The Unchained Spirit

Or, the glass is half-full, but I've forgotten where I put it

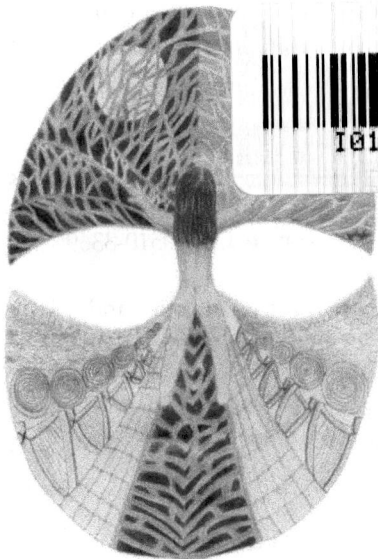

Barbara Lieberman

This book is not intended as a substitute for the medical advice of physicians and licensed professionals. The reader should regularly consult a physician and/or certified health practitioners in matters relating to his/her health and particularly with respect to any symptoms that may require diagnosis or medical attention. The author is not liable if the reader relies upon the material and is injured in some way. Where the author's personal memories are cited, the recollection of stories shared are recalled to the best of the author's knowledge.

A Pipe & Thimble Publishing Book
PO Box 3369
Torrance, CA 90510-3369

Original art for front cover and title page
by Barbara Lieberman
Copyright © 2006, 2016. All rights reserved.
Back cover photo of the author and her hand-carved
walking stick, soon after she began walking in 2006.

First edition.

ISBN-13: 978-0692783108
ISBN-10: 0692783105

Books by Barbara Lieberman:

The Treasure of Ravenwood: A Fairy Tale
To Miss the Stars
Message on the Wind (Book 1 of the McEwen Series)
To Reap a Whirlwind (Book 2 of the McEwen Series)
Dragonmarsh: A Horde of Dragons Anthology
Unchaining Your Spirit: Living with Chronic Illness

Illustrated Children's Books:
Ben's Little Acorn
Ben's Little Acorn Coloring Activity Book
Why Does the Moon Follow Me?
Why Does the Moon Follow Me? Coloring Activity Book

Table of Contents

FOREWORD I

ACKNOWLEDGEMENTS v

"HELLO, MY NAME IS BARB AND I'M FINE" 1

THE MONSTER IN THE CLOSET 5

RIDING THE WAVES 11

Denial 12

Anger 14

Bargaining 16

Depression 17

Acceptance 19

Getting stuck 20

Why me? 23

TAKING CONTROL 25

Food 27

   Going Raw 29

Mindful Eating 38

Meditation 41

Visualization 48

Get moving 50

   Walking 52

   Swimming and water work 53

   Other methods 54

Flower pots 57

Cry when you need to 59

Rest 59

Inner Work 61

Then sings my soul... 66

Faith 68

FRIENDS — ANCHORS, LIFELINES, AND SPOONS 71

Lifelines 71

Borrowing spoons 73

INTIMACY, RELATIONSHIPS, AND ILLNESS 77

MAKING LEMONADE 83

Creative outlets 83

Art as Healing   86
Finding joy   94
Build a community   96
Find your gifts   97
Humor   98

WHEN YOU CARE ABOUT SOMEONE WITH A CHRONIC

ILLNESS...   101
The New Normal: Holding Space   102
Helping isn't always helpful   105
Sticks and Stones...the power of words   107
Caregivers – the unsung heroes   109
Shut up and dance with me   113
When you don't hear from me   115
Little things add up   115

ADVOCACY AND SUPPORT   117
When you ask for help   119
  When the answer is yes: 120
  When the answer is no: 120

ADAPTING TO CHANGE, AND LIVING VERSUS EXISTING

                                                                123
Life, written in pencil   124
Learn to say 'no'   125
Learn to say 'maybe'   127
Learn to say 'yes'! New ways to do old things   128
Learn to say 'yes': new things   130
Make the most of the good days, self-care on the bad days 132
The internet as a lifeline   133
"Morning song"   135
Tools of the trade   137
  Covering the cost   140
  Another thought   140

TO TELL OR NOT TO TELL...   143

THE GIFT OF CHRONIC ILLNESS   147

AFTER THE MIRACLE   151
"Survivor" to "Phoenix"   154

TANGIBLE ADVICE AT A GLANCE   157

WHEN THE RUG IS PULLED OUT FROM UNDER YOU...

LIVING UNDIAGNOSED   161

THIS GLORIOUS LIFE   167

LIVING OUR TRUTH   177

EPILOGUE: MONSTER SLAYER   183

APPENDICES   185

Recipes to get you started   **185**

Kitchen add-ons: **188**

  Nutty for Nut Milk   190

  Gratifying Granola   191

  Mouth-watering Miso Soup   192

  Garden-fresh Gazpacho   193

  Dressing to impress   194

  Hummus to Hum About   195

  Hummus Revisited   196

  It's Better Raw Salsa   197

  Fabulous Flax Crackers   198

  Scrumptious Salmon Salad   199

  You Can Have Your "Pasta" Too (single serving) 200

  Pesto Sauce   200

  Tomato Sauce   200

  Tantalizing Raw Tacos   202

  Start Your Day Right Toast   203

  Barb's Baba Ganoush   204

  Power Breakfast   205

  Personal Care Recipes   207

  Radiant Skin Scrub   208

  Worry-free Antiperspirant   209

Other books and websites to help you get started   **210**

  Referenced books: 210

  Raw Food Diet and Overcoming Illness with Food 210

  Growing and Using Herbs   211

  Meditation, Visualization, Celtic Spirituality, Ecopsychology,
  and Reconnecting with the Earth   211

  Shamanism and Soul-Retrieval   212

  Art as Healing   213

Websites: 214

ABOUT THE AUTHOR
UNCHAINING YOUR SPIRIT

Foreword

When Barbara asked me to write the foreword for *The Unchained Spirit*, I was deeply honored and emotionally touched by her outreach. When we spoke, she said she had reached out to me because it just "felt right" and, together, we assumed our connection was as a result of our similar beliefs in the power of food as healing, my knowledge of such, and my experience in developing healing, healthy recipes.

When I learned of her work, I gladly accepted not knowing then what the true connection would ultimately turn out to be. While we share the connection of food as healing, we also share the journey of chronic illness. For me, the journey is not as the frustrated patient but as one of a team of family and friend caregivers.

My mother-in-law was diagnosed with Stage 4 Ovarian Cancer in 2015. You will come to reflect on the theory of "stages" as you read *The Unchained Spirit* but, as modern science categorizes chronic illness, my mother-in-law's diagnosis was severe. And out of the blue. This diagnosis came as a shock to the family because just the year before she had undergone surgery to remove the possibility of cancer and was told she was cancer-free.

At the time of the diagnosis, she was given seven days to live. Family flew in to say their goodbyes. We all thought it was the end. Yet, her partner, Debbie, and son, Chris, saw some spark in her and, while still in the hospital, she became stronger. She looked her oncologist in the eye and said, "I am not ready to die. I am going to beat this."

Against the odds, Lois went home on hospice at

first. Nutrition bags, power ports, pain medications, G-tubes... these all became terms we got to know very quickly. Debbie took time off of work to care for her daily. Friends and family were placed on duty around the clock.

Miracles happened, and Lois lived what most would call a normal life. She had her "bag" she carried with her for her G-tube and together they went... on a drive through the neighborhoods during the holidays to view the Christmas lights, to her favorite casinos, fishing, and to the beach with her grand-niece and -nephew.

Lois saw her granddaughter graduate from high school and head off to college. She lived many full, vibrant days in between chemotherapy treatments, hospitalized bouts of dehydration, infection, pneumonia, exhaustion, and nausea. All of this was made possible by her faith in God, her strong will to live, and the dedication of her caregivers.

Every word Barbara writes is so true. She says:
"My truth is different than yours."
".... Children need to be children..."
".... Caregivers need at least as much support as clients do."
"Grief comes in waves."

Riding the waves, Denial, Anger, Bargaining, Depression, Acceptance, Taking Control, Food, Exercise, Community, Advocacy and Support... Barbara connects the base realities with an understanding of the emotion behind it, for both the affected and the ones caring for the affected: the patient and the caregivers. She has created a step-by-step guide to what to expect when faced with a chronic illness and from many points of view. From how you are going to feel emotionally, to the physical challenges, the relational difficulties, her written words are so eloquent that you feel uplifted, encouraged and privileged to have gained such knowledge.

As a Certified Food Healer and Fitness Nutritionist, I encourage you to dive in to the food and exercise sections of the book. Food is medicine... both good and bad. It is up to each individual to learn as much as they can about their health condition and take seriously the foods that can help heal them either partially or fully or to just relieve symptoms. Food matters. What you eat daily matters. What you put in to your body daily makes all the difference in the quality of your health. It does. I implore you to take your health seriously.

At the time of this writing, Lois is in her final days. It is my firm belief that she lived fully beyond those "seven days to live" because of her faith in God, her loving caregivers, her change in diet, and, mostly, her desire to live.

Everyone should read *The Unchained Spirit*. Doing so will help you gain awareness into a territory unseen, a path unknown in what to expect with a chronic illness both for the patient and for the caregivers. Knowledge is strength and strength is healing... both of which everyone will need in these steps of life. This book is a powerful guidebook even for those who are not ill, as chances are a family member or a friend or friend of a friend is struggling to understanding a chronic health condition either now or will be in the future. The patient, the caregivers... family, close friends, nurses, doctors, everyone will receive new light in understanding how chronic illness impacts many lives in a multitude of ways.

For Lois' care, I would like to share that her

primary caregiver, Debbie, fought hard for her and endured much financial, emotional, and physical sacrifice. We are all grateful, Debbie, for your love, diligence and sacrifice during the last two years. We express gratitude for Lois' sister, Margie, her son, Chris, and so many loving friends and dear neighbors for their care and dedication to Lois' healing. There can be joy and hope in living with chronic illness. Barbara gives you great direct insight in to how.

- Susan Irby, creator of The Bikini Chef®

About the author: Susan Irby is certified in Fitness Nutrition and Food Healing. An award-winning author, television host and radio personality, Susan is the creator of the *The Bikini Chef*® brand, its recipes and content. *The Bikini Chef*® promotes "figure flattering flavors" and living a healthy lifestyle through good nutrition, delicious foods, and fitness. Currently, Susan is the Chef behind the recipes in Dr. Ward Bond and Chef Susan Irby *Healing Remedies & Recipes* online class. Dr. Bond and Susan have a television show in development. She is also the creator, producer, and former host of *The Bikini Lifestyles*® *Show* and is author of nine books on cooking and wellness. Visit **healingremediesandrecipes.com** for show and class information.

www.susanirby.com
Facebook/thebikinichef
Twitter/@TheSusanIrby   **Twitter/thebikinichef**
 Instagram/thebikinichef   **Instagram/thesusanirby**
 Contact Susan at: (310) 753-3750 or email: susan@susanirby.com

ACKNOWLEDGMENTS

This book would not have been possible without the following people:

My children, Ben and Ellie Lieberman, who give me strength when I have none, courage when I falter, and love always;

Beta readers, heart friends, and Tribe members Ellie Lieberman, Evangeline Duran Fuentes, and Robin Nieto, who offered so much perspective, support, and enthusiasm for this project;

My talented, artistic and generous friend, Jessica Johnson, who said 'yes, the time is now' to publishing this book;

Susan Irby, creator of The Bikini Chef®, for her support and belief in this project;

And, my parents, Richard and Marguerite Austin, who walked their talk and taught me to live with courage, faith, and love. I owe them this glorious life.

This book is dedicated to all who live with
chronic illness and pain…
May your Spirit always fly free!

"Hello, my name is Barb and I'm fine"

This is a very different book than the one I first set out to write nine years ago. I started writing that book to celebrate my new life in remission, completely symptom-free. I was walking again, driving again, and saw no signs of the monster in the closet. It was a book to not only celebrate that, but also to share ways toward health and healing for others.

Here I am, a decade later, publishing a very different book. I have relapsed again after nine symptom-free years. I am facing many of the same challenges of the past and some new ones this time around. I am still fighting, still refusing to let illness take over my body and my life. As a result, I am sharing a very different book with you.

Living with a chronic illness is sort of like having a stranger move into your house, uninvited and unwelcome. You can give up and just blame everything on the stranger, or you can work with it and around it to create a life in spite of the intrusion.

It's not unlike saying you have faith but blaming your lack of motivation on the devil. "Well, I would do more (or better), but the devil keeps knocking me down." It's up to us to knock our devil, our illness, down.

I fight every single day to appear 'normal,' to feel 'normal', to pretend to be 'fine'. You may not realize just how much that can cost me, in strength and energy. If you feel there is a disconnect between that and 'the truth', there most certainly is, and I'm living it every single day. That is what chronic illness is... a disconnect between what our souls can do and what our bodies can do.

My truth is different than yours. The simplest things are a struggle, yet I will fiercely defend my right to do them... and to fall down, topple over, lose sleep, and hurt myself in the process. If you love me, let me do what I must and hear me when I ask for help, even when it's a mere whisper.

Please don't tell me not to overdo, not to do too much, and not to give up. Don't wax poetic about how strong I am, and how great I look in spite of everything. I'm truly happy that I inspire you, but I rarely *feel* inspiring. While you may think I'm brave, to me there is no other choice but to plow through, forge ahead, and keep going.

There are days when showering is a challenge. There are days when I have to double-check that I've put on all my clothes and my shoes, before I go out. There are days when the fatigue is so great, I have to think about heading to the bathroom before I actually get up the nerve to give it a shot.

On the other hand, there are days when I feel better, clearer, brighter. I cherish those days and overdo it on those days, and you have to let me. I will not heed your warning to take it easy, to reserve my strength, and to 'be careful'. I don't want to be careful. As a character in my story *Love in the Middle* says, "I want to be bold and reckless and go where my spirit takes me. Don't you?"

In between, there are days when my body is not cooperating, but my spirit is soaring. The experience of writing this book was made up of just such days. And, I continue to soar. It is my wish that you will soar alongside me.

The Monster in the Closet

On October 12, 2006, I placed my hands on the arms of my chair, my feet flat on the ground, and pushed myself up to stand. That may not seem like something miraculous and, yet, it was a life-changing moment. The chair was a wheelchair, and it had been almost nine years since I'd stood on my own.

What feat lasted only a few seconds, but it was the beginning of a new life for me and the end of an era. By the end of that month, I was walking, albeit it with assistance. Today, I am still walking, dancing a little, and still struggling.

Living with a chronic illness is like living with a monster in the closet. The monster doesn't only haunt the person who is ill. It also haunts all those who live with and care about that person.

My children used to leave for school every day wondering whether I would be able to walk, speak, or move my arms when they got home. They were constantly afraid I would have a seizure and, despite my best efforts to reassure them otherwise, that illness would rob them of me forever.

The following is a speech I gave to a very special group of people...WAMS or Women Against MS... in the Spring of 2006. In it, I explained all this from my own perspective:

I am 44 and proud of it. I am an authentic redhead, not a natural one. I am the mother of two amazing children. I am a sister. I love to garden and to read and I am an aspiring novelist. I love old television westerns and I still love Monty Python. I am a long-suffering Phillies fan and I loved curling long before this Olympics.

I also have Multiple Sclerosis. I don't mind talking about my MS. But, I don't really like to talk about how I feel and I usually make incredibly tasteless jokes about incontinence and Depends at this point in the conversation. There are so many other things I'd rather do than tell you that I have no sensation but pain from the neck down. That I have deep neuromuscular pain, allodynia and photophobia and I have no sense of hunger or other functions in my body. That I have weakness in my arms. That I suffer seizures that rob me of my speech for days. That I have not walked in almost eight years. That my memory is sporadic, on good days, non-existent on bad ones and that I suffer from intense sensory overload.

Misdiagnosed since the early 1980's, my symptoms finally got a name in 2000. A diagnosis of MS meant for me finally putting a name to my adversary, a face to the beast. I fight better when I know what I'm fighting. After all, no one fights well in the dark.

But, MS isn't about myelin or lesions when you have it. MS is that monster in the darkness you feared in childhood. Sometimes, it hid in the closet. Sometimes, it waited under the bed. It had no face but you knew it was there. No one ever believed you. No one else could see it. But, you knew it was there...waiting for you each and every time your mom or dad turned out the light. I have no idea what it will look like tonight, tomorrow, or the next day. But, I always know it's there.

Having MS means not knowing if the right word will come out of my mouth, if I can think of a word at all. It means not riding amusements with my kids, not tucking them in at night, not cooking if I'm alone. It means not driving my son to baseball practice or picking my daughter up from a sleepover. It means not walking my kids home from the bus stop. It means being afraid to venture away from home alone, for fear a seizure will render me completely and utterly helpless.

But, believe it or not, it has also been a gift, or as I like to say 'the glass is half full. I

just can't remember where I put it.'
Unfortunately, I can't exchange or return this
particular gift.

My MS gave me two years of spending
almost every day with my parents before I lost
them both suddenly four years ago. It has
shown me I am not really in control of
anything. It has taught me to relinquish worry
and fear, because these just exhaust me while
serving no real purpose. It has brought new
activities into my life, to fill the holes left by old
ones I can no longer do. And, it has brought
wonderful, unforgettable people into my circle
of friends.

MS has allowed me to teach my children
that you love someone no matter what happens
to them. They've seen that they can face
anything and overcome it. They've seen that
disability means nothing and that accessibility
simply means finding new ways to do old
things. And, yes, we've learned to laugh in the
face of the monster.

Having support has helped us do just
that. I have never ceased to be amazed by the
wonderful people at groups like the National
MS Society. I have never once called a single
person on the staff who did not help me,
support me or answer my questions. They own
every phone call. They carry my family on their
broad shoulders, through the mire of this
untenable illness. They remember that my
children need to be children, despite this illness

of mine. They remember that caregivers need at least as much support as clients do. How can you help but be impressed by people who are working so hard to put themselves out of a job?

What I want you to know is that no one person has MS. There are not 400,000 people with MS in the US or 11,000 people here with it in the Delaware Valley. When I left the Dr. office with MS, so did my parents, my children and my siblings. So did my neighbors, my church congregation and every other person who knows and cares about me.

There are millions of us with MS. Millions of us who suffer its effects. Millions waiting and hoping and working toward a cure. Those millions of people know that MS changes the lives of every person it touches. Those millions know that MS is a monster waiting in the dark. But, surely, if millions speak, someone will believe us. And, surely, if there are millions of us, we can turn on the light and slay this monster once and for all.

There are many different chronic illnesses, life-threatening diseases, and long-term physical and mental challenges that can present themselves at our doorstep at any given moment. While my perspective is shared from my own journey, this book addresses what many of us face every single day, whether you are the one living with the illness/disease or you are someone who loves a person so challenged.

Riding the waves

With all due respect to Elizabeth Kubler-Ross, I've always felt that calling what we experience when faced with a loved one's death or diagnosed with a chronic illness 'stages' makes them sound simple, manageable, and finite. It's as if you're going to be standing there, waiting for a train. You board at stage one and ride to the next stop. There, you get off and get on the next train for the next 'stage' of your grief. But, grieving is not simple, it's not easy, and it doesn't come in simple, straightforward stages. It also knows no set time frame.

Grief comes in waves. Big, scary, often unanticipated waves that can knock you down and make you feel as if you're drowning. Those waves can come straight for you, or from the side when you're not looking. Often, the different waves take turns; sometimes, they join forces. And, then, there's the undertow. It can pull you under and out to sea before you even realize you've left the safety of the shoreline. It can set you adrift, feeling as if you have no lifeline or anchor.

Why am I writing about grief? Because when you're diagnosed with a chronic or life-threatening illness, you're going to grieve. If you accept this premise up front, you can wax up your board and expect the unexpected. Being aware of what's coming is the best weapon in your arsenal.

The stages are a handy tool, for identifying what you're feeling and why, as far as tools go. They are sort of like that ridiculous pain scale. Ever try to put a number on your pain? Yeah, I hate that one. The stages serve a purpose, but can also make you feel as if you're stuck or failing if you don't recognize their limitations. So, let's take a look at them...

Denial

Yeah, we've been there, right? This isn't happening to me. They made a mistake. I don't have _____ (fill in your diagnosis). Or, if you're like me, I actually welcomed the correct diagnosis. Not because it was good news, but because it was news.

As I've written elsewhere, it's easier for me to fight if I know what I'm fighting. With a diagnosis like, relapsing/remitting MS, the denial came after a nine-year remission. The presenting symptoms the third time around were different, and it took a while for it to "look like" MS (more on this later in the book).

I didn't want to believe it was MS. First, I didn't want to believe it could come back. Second, someone in my life had made it pretty clear that if the MS moved in, he would move out. See, there is a lot that goes into these stages and not all of it comes from within us.

Perhaps you are in denial because you've read marriage statistics for MS or other chronic illness. Perhaps you're in denial because you fear losing your job. Whatever the reason, the sooner you accept your diagnosis, the sooner you can get busy fighting your battle.

That pesky Pain Scale can be a place of denial for those of us living with chronic illness, chronic pain, and/or life-threatening diseases. Doctors love methods of assessing where we are in any given moment and this is one of those handy tools they use. Unfortunately, we tend to lie, on one hand; we tend to deny, on the other.

Yes, we lie. 'I'm fine' being the main lie but lowering our pain rating is a way we deny just how badly we're feeling. If we deny it, we can push through it and avoiding 'giving in'.

I remember in *The Fault in Our Stars* by John Green, when Hazel Grace offered a nine on the pain scale when asked, because she was saving her ten. I related to so much in that movie, even at my age, but that line struck at my soul.

I always save my tens. When the pain was so unbearable that no scale could measure it, I still offered nine as my response.

This is one area where denial can really take a toll. You try to continue to live as you always have, and deny your body and soul what they need. I'm not talking about prescription pain medications, though they may be an option for you. I'm referring more to ways of taking care of yourself when you feel really awful. Admitting that you feel really awful is the first step. Then, letting your body and soul tell you what they need, and you listening, is the next. It's not selfish; it's self-preservation.

Rest, time outdoors in fresh air and your toes in the grass or sand, darkness and silence, a serious snuggle from your partner, a long scented bath, prayer, meditation, counseling, immersing yourself in your favorite music, savoring a delicious, beautiful meal... allow yourself these prescriptions too. They are no less important to your journey and your well-being.

Anger

Well, hell, yes, I'm angry. I'm angry that it took so long to diagnose me initially, wasting precious years of treatment. I'm angry that it keeps coming back, when I think it's been long gone. I'm angry at my body for betraying me, and at life partners who can't handle it. I'm angry at an inaccessible world, when we should have long ago made the world a place we can all live in. I'm angry with a medical community that cannot make up its mind. That's a lot of anger.

Anger is a natural, healthy reaction to what life throws at us. It can be a very motivating feeling, so you have to let yourself be angry. You may have been brought up to believe that nice people don't get angry. Patently untrue and very harmful, when you spend all your energy suppressing what you truly feel.

It is my personal belief that a lot of what we manifest physically is triggered by what we repress emotionally. Healthy anger can spur you to seek better treatment or to change your diet. It can open your eyes to unhealthy, toxic relationships. But, like all the stages, it is somewhere you can get stuck. And getting stuck here will get you mired down in the muck with no forward movement.

One thing that really helps is being angry at the right things. It may take a bit of poking around in your psyche to figure out the root or roots of your anger, but this effort goes a long way to helping you face it, learn from it, and move on.

Think of it as pulling up dandelions. It's easy to yank on that flower above the grass, and it will come out with some small roots. But, the long tap roots are the real problem and require a lot more digging to truly get to the bottom of them.

Too often, we strike out at our closest contacts, usually the one who is our caregiver, partner or best friend, and use them as a whipping post. This may seem natural to do; they love us no matter what, right? This not only wounds and confuses them, it also prevents us from having to go within to find the culprit. So, deflecting is definitely not the answer.

This is where counseling can be a huge help. You can say anything to a counselor, but they can call you on your bullshit. That may be hard to hear, at first, but it allows you to get the anger out of your body, without hurting anyone else's feelings, while getting real, effective feedback on where you are emotionally and get the help you need to stay on track.

Bargaining

There isn't a lot of bargaining in chronic illness. At least, in my experience there isn't. But, if you blame yourself for what's happening to you, or if you blame some outside force for handing you this pile of crap, you very well may find yourself thinking "if I do x, then y will surely happen" or "Ok, God, you got me. I'll do better. Learned my lesson. So, you can take this away now". All of this only serves to hold you back.

To move forward, we have to accept that this illness is here, now, in this moment. But, so are many opportunities masked as challenges. If you find yourself thinking "If only…" try and determine what it is you are avoiding in that moment. Hold the spotlight there, as uncomfortable as that may be, and work on that.

Depression

When I first received the diagnosis of MS, the doctor handed me a pile of prescriptions and an appointment card for three months in the future. That was all I received, at that point. I couldn't help but notice that one of the prescriptions was for an antidepressant. When I asked him why he'd given me that, he replied that I was depressed and it would help me cope. I argued that I wasn't depressed. His point was that I had to be. Any sane person would be, right?

Really? Has it come to that? Do we just assume we're all depressed now? Because, quite honestly, I wasn't. I could clearly identify that I was angry it had taken so long to get my diagnosis right. That I was relieved to finally have the correct diagnosis and could now fight what was happening to me. That I was frightened of what could still yet happen. But, depressed? Nope.

This is not to say that I have not experienced situational depression at any point. I will not say that my third relapse did not hit me hard. I also will not say it hasn't depressed me. Depression happens no matter how well-adjusted we are. This is also not to say that no one should ever take an antidepressant. This is to say, however, that we need health practitioners who will tailor our treatments to us as individuals.

My most recent counselor asked questions to determine if I was experiencing depression, as my relapse was confirmed. These include 'are you having trouble sleeping?' Have my eating habits changed? Do I feel any sense of pleasure or joy on a daily basis? Even then, if she felt that I was experiencing depression, she discussed all the options for dealing with it. My current neurologist asked the same things, to determine if antidepressants were appropriate.

When experiencing depression, whether or not you decide to take medication, do find a trustworthy person to speak with. Licensed clinical social workers and other licensed counselors can help you by listening to you, allowing you to cry and rant in a safe space, and give you exercises to help you work through it.

It is also important to remember that you are in control of your treatment. If you feel your counselor is not a good fit for you, ask for a different one. It will not hurt his/her feelings, but it will get you the help you need. It is your right to find the best fit for you.

It is essential that if you feel like hurting yourself, taking your life, or hurting someone else, that you reach out for help. The situation may feel hopeless, but I am living proof it is not. Help is there and you need to reach for it. And if someone you love is saying they don't want to live, take them seriously and seek help for them. We don't always know the right words to express our despair, so listen carefully and take no chances with someone else's well-being.

Asking questions does not spur someone to action. Avoidance might. If someone you love is saying, "I don't want to do this anymore" or "I don't want to live like this", ask the question "are you saying you want to kill yourself?" Ask! The answer is important and, if the answer is anything other than a firm 'NO!', then please seek help in dealing with the situation. People who are suicidal are in a place that does not allow for thinking clearly. They don't consider how you will feel about it, because they can't. Outside intervention is essential to save their lives.

Acceptance

Acceptance is not giving in. Let me say that again, acceptance is not giving in. Because, hear me now, I will never, ever give in to my illness. I will fight it with every breath I take, every step I take, and every moment I have.

What acceptance does mean is that I have an illness and it is a part of this package I call 'me' now. It's along for the ride. I can't shake it anymore than I can my surgery scars (yet), but, having accepted it is here, I can adapt, adjust, and accommodate where and when I have to... and keep going. There is just a 'new normal' for me, and for you.

When we accept that we have a chronic illness, we can also accept the treatments for it. We can begin to focus on doing the things we need to live life to the fullest and to keep as healthy as we can, despite our challenges. Notice again, there is no 'giving in' or 'giving up'. There is simply 'living with'.

I'd also like to add that I never use the phrase "I suffer from my illness". I do often suffer from its effects. However, the moment "I suffer from X" becomes part of your vocabulary and your self-description, you lose control of it. You empower the monster, not the other way around.

You live with illness, yes. I have red hair and I have an illness. They are both part of what makes me 'me', at least for now. But, please don't use "I suffer from X" because, as I repeat often, thoughts become things (tut.com). I have an illness, but it doesn't have me.

Getting stuck

I mentioned this before, but it is worth looking at even more closely. It is not uncommon that we get stuck in one of the stages of grief, whether triggered by chronic illness or the loss of a loved one. It is important to have real lifelines in your journey, for when the waves of emotions knock you over. Those who know us best often recognize that we're stuck long before we do. We need people to tell us what they see happening. We need people we can hold on to. And, we need to hear them when they do.

Talking is the best way to work out where we are and what we're feeling. Talking to your spouse, parent, or child, however, can be fraught with minefields. Do you really want to tell your wife you feel all alone in this? Do you want to lay your fears on your child's shoulders? This is when a counselor or support group can be your lifeline: a group of people, facing what you are facing but not necessarily in love with you or relying on you. A good counselor who will listen, poke what you avoid, and call bullshit when you need to hear it, can be exactly what you need to face down your demons.

Just be sure to find the right fit. You have the right to ask for a different counselor, if the one you're seeing isn't the one who can do the most good. You have the right to leave a group whenever you feel the time is right. Know your rights, do your homework, but find an outlet for yourself.

All of this can be a very difficult thing to process through and accept. It comes in waves, because what we face changes from day to day.

Just when you think 'I've got this', your body goes 'nope, here's a new challenge for ya!'

It's also difficult because we find ourselves not only coping with our own feelings, our own 'waves' of emotion, but those of others, as we explain what has happened and what has changed. Try to remember that you are not responsible for how other people react nor how they perceive your illness and how you are coping with it. You can only control your own response and your own reactions.

Likewise, if someone you love is coping with a life-changing illness, you have your own set of feelings and stages to go through. Yes, things are going to change for you, too, and you need to find your own 'new normal'. You have the right to every stage of grief, and you, too, need to find a healthy, supportive outlet where you can express those feelings and deal with them.

One word, okay maybe more than one, about men, women, and talking. Women, in general, have been taught to express our feelings more openly since we are young. That is not to say that we all do this, or that this is true in every instance. I have had my own issues of holding in my feelings to protect others from them.

My mother, for example, suffered greatly over my birth defect. I tried hard not to show her my pain or cry in front of her as a result. That has led to a feeling that when I do need to release those feelings, it must be done in private, rather than to distress others or lay my pain on their shoulders.

But, men, particularly those who are now middle-aged or older, were not taught to honor their feelings or put them into words. The vulnerability of doing so can be ego-shattering; not to mention the whole 'crying makes you a girl' attitude. The process of starting to talk these things out can be very, very difficult. But, it is well worth it.

The truth is that it is not a sign of weakness to seek out a counselor. It is a sign of strength, an act of courage. To open up and reveal ourselves to another, in order to cope with all we face, is yet another prescription we need and one we owe ourselves to fill.

Why me?

Are you asking this? This is one place we can get stuck, and it's a tough one to climb out of. Why isn't prayer working for me? Why do others seem to cope better than I do? Why is this happening to me? Why can't I get answers? Why can't I get any relief?

These are all valid questions, and it is normal to ask them and to feel the accompanying anger and frustration. On the other hand, it is focusing us in the wrong direction if we want to really live, versus existing.

What do I mean by that?

Focusing on why things aren't working, or why you aren't getting well, means you're not focusing on what you *can* still do and what *is* working for you. It's not focusing on changing what you can, and on being in control of the things you still can control. This is true any time you focus on lack, rather than on possibility.

Try flipping your thoughts, when the 'why?' starts. I've found that it helps me to think in terms of 'what can I do?' rather than 'why can't I do this?' And, the powerful 'why not?' when thinking of ways to feel better and do more. 'Why not' eat better; what do I have to lose'? 'Why not try exercising'? 'Why not create something beautiful... or try something new... or give that dream a chance'?

Flip the 'whys' and give yourself a shot at really living your life. Fill that prescription!

Taking control

You may have seen a quote from the late Wayne Dyer, that when we change the way we look at things, the things we look at change. It is amazing how one seemingly small decision can change everything in the space of one moment. It is important that those decisions are yours.

During my second relapse, I experienced intense, unrelenting pain over my entire body. When touched, I felt as if thousands of burning razor blades were being raked across my skin. I couldn't bear to be touched by my children, my clothing, the shower, or even a breeze.

After consulting a local pain specialist, I underwent two in-hospital intrathecal trials. This involved inserting a catheter into my spinal fluid and then testing different pain medications, in different combinations, to see if any would relieve my pain. While Demerol® did ease my pain, it also dangerously suppressed my respiration and so was not a viable choice.

Finally, a combination of drugs was selected and an intrathecal pump (think metal hockey puck) installed into my abdomen.

Within two months of the surgery, my feet began to swell. Though there was no indication in any documentation that the combination of drugs in my pump would cause swelling, swell they did. In fact, I had no ankles and the pressure in my already pained legs was unbearable.

To make matters worse, a vascular surgeon prescribed treatment with pressure boots to relieve the swelling. That meant I was to put on long plastic boots, covering my feet and legs up to my knees, and have air pumped into the boots to compress my swollen legs. It was, quite literally, torture. I cried through every treatment. So did my children.

The treatment to relieve the swelling caused by the drugs to relieve the pain did not work. One year after the pump was installed, and the pain continually worsened, I was in danger of losing one of my feet. Finally, the pump was removed at my insistence. The very next day, I had ankles and all traces of swelling were gone. So much for no interaction between the drugs. I was back to square one but in even more pain than I had been the year before. Again, there seemed no solution.

What was important was that I spoke up and followed my instincts. I knew what was causing the problem and, despite all those who said otherwise, I insisted the pump be removed and the meds stopped. And, I was right.

I am not saying you should never listen to doctors or others who are participating in your care. In fact, I'm saying the exact opposite: you *should* listen, attentively, carefully, and ask a lot of questions. You should read and research and learn all you can. And, then, you should take the course of action that makes sense for you.

Food

Let food be thy medicine, thy medicine shall be thy food. - Hippocrates

There some areas of your life where you can immediately take control, for your own good. One is food and meals. This is an area of your life that can either contribute to health or contribute to sickness. It's all up to you.

Take a careful look at your average supermarket and you will probably discover that the best food for you is around the perimeter. The more central the aisles, the more processed the food. Some food chains are changing for the better, stocking more and more nutritious and healthy choices, but one thing is absolutely certain. You need to read labels.

The further removed a food is from its original form, the less good it can do you. Add in salt and sugar and hydrogenated oils and long, unpronounceable chemical ingredients, and you will do more harm than good. There are so many healthier things to eat. And, thankfully, supermarkets are taking advantage of the general public's desire to do just that.

Now, you can get packs of fresh fruit, cheese, nuts to snack on. You can get granola instead of sugared cereals. There are entire rows of organic items to choose from. Other market chains specialize in raw, organic, chemical-free, free-range, wild harvested food choices. There are some challenges to eating this way, one being that the food doesn't keep as long and, so, you have to shop more frequently. However, the advantages outweigh the disadvantages beyond count.

One rule I've heard is not to eat anything you cannot pronounce. Another is to not eat anything ants won't touch, margarine being one example. For me, I stick with the 'as close to nature' rule whenever possible. I eat raw as often as possible. I eat low-fat as often as possible, and choose fats carefully. I eat as many servings of fruit and vegetables a day as possible. I drink filtered water as often as possible.

On the flip side, I avoid fast foot, soda, packaged/processed foods and processed meats, refined sugars, and refined grains as often as possible. Notice, I do not say that I *never* eat these things. And, that brings me to another point about food.

Eating is not only good for your body; it's good for your soul. Sometimes, you need a piece of smooth, sweet chocolate. Sometimes, a piece of fried chicken is just the ticket. Sometimes, you crave that ranch chip. I love grilled cheddar cheese sandwiches with fresh basil leaves. I say, eat 'em (unless there is a very good reason not to, such as diabetes).

A little bit will soothe a craving and soothe your soul. Ignore the craving and you'll find yourself at the bottom of a box of store-bought cookies wondering how you got there. Then, you'll throw up your hands in defeat and throw out the whole plan.

Instead, think of the big picture. A week of healthy eating and then one candy bar is not going to break you. Just pay attention to why you're making the choice you are and, then, enjoy it. Savor it. And, go back to eating well.

Going Raw

"You pray for good health and a body that will be strong in old age. Good — but your rich foods block the gods' answer and tie Jupiter's hands." Persivs Satvrae II.41-43

I am the first to admit this is something I would never have tried years ago. Quite honestly, years ago, it would have been a great deal more difficult. Thanks to places like Trader Joe's™, Whole Foods™, Sprouts™, and local markets going organic and, suddenly, eating raw is a great deal easier than it used to be. The selections these markets offer, supplemented by your own local farmer's markets, make going raw a viable option.

Supporting your local farmers also adds to your local economy and means you're not paying high transportation costs on top of the price of the food, while improving your own health. Can't find what you want? Ask your supermarket produce manager to carry more organic produce and then be sure to purchase it when he or she complies with your request.

You'll note here that I said 'easier'. This is not an easy regimen to follow. It involves careful shopping and daily preparation of your meals (because your food has no preservatives), and shopping more frequently because fresh, organic, raw food requires extra trips to the market for whatever you don't grow yourself.

It means knowing what restaurants serve before you go, and packing lunch and snacks for work. You must be constantly aware of what you are putting in your mouth and what it does for and to your body. That is the point of the exercise, after all.

In some ways, however, it is less work. Think about it… you prepare the food, but you don't cook it. You save time. You save effort. You save energy costs. More shopping, less steps of food preparation.

The reason for eating raw is because cooking destroys the very enzymes that benefit us. Enzymes, like proteins, are vulnerable to heat. Vitamins like Vitamin C and folic acid, along with enzymes and proteins, are literally destroyed by cooking them at temperatures about 106-107 degrees.

Calcium is not absorbed as well at higher temperatures. Calcium in raw milk is absorbed more easily into your body than calcium from milk that has been pasteurized. Oxalic acid from cooked spinach has been linked to kidney stones, while the oxalic acid from raw spinach is more easily absorbed into your body.

Other foods, such as beans and nuts, do not release their energy unless they are germinated and/or sprouted. This allows the enzymes to be released, because their natural inhibitors are neutralized. You get both the protein and the enzymes, unlike what you get with cooked beans or nuts or non-germinated raw ones.

Juicing is important because certain vegetables and fruits, carrots for example, require their cellular structure to be broken down before you can receive their full benefits. Munching on a raw carrot will not give you the full benefits of its beta-carotene, along with the enzymes. Juicing is the only way to get both. Just be sure to drink the juice as soon as you prepare it if you have a centrifugal juicer, or it will begin to oxidize and lose its benefits.

With a raw-food lifestyle, I can eat whatever I want, whenever I want it. There is no measuring, portioning or weighing. I eat smaller meals more often and enjoy every one of them. I snack between meals with no guilt. I never feel deprived or feel as if I'm dieting.

This last point is important. Whenever you decide to 'go on a diet', you are already thinking of how you can deprive yourself of 'bad' food, for some end goal. That is exactly why diets don't work. Instead, look to change your lifestyle. Consider eating to feel and look better, rather than giving up what you love.

Visit those sections of the produce department or the farmer's market that you've never ventured into before. Pick up jicama or bok choy and give them a try. There is a world of foods that we haven't tasted, and it can become an exciting adventure to do just that.

We can also address specific symptoms with food choices. I suffer terribly from summer's high temperatures, for example. Maybe you are experiencing hot flashes from menopause. Well, juice a couple of raw cucumbers and pour that over some ice, for an amazingly easy, natural, raw way to feel cooler. Or add raw cucumbers and peppermint leaves to your water bottle, to infuse it with cooling goodness.

In her book, *Eating in the Raw*, Carol Alt suggests deciding first exactly what foods you cannot live without. Then, see if that food has a raw 'twin' or much-healthier alternative, something you can substitute to satisfy that craving. For me, that wasn't necessary, as I wasn't eating much to begin with the first time around. For you, it may be essential.

If you absolutely must have pasta, try a recipe the recipe in this book for spiral-cut squash and raw tomato sauce. If cheese is your comfort food, try raw milk cheeses. Stores like Whole Foods™ and Trader Joe's™ have a great selection of raw cow, goat, and sheep's milk cheeses, and mine is staffed with friendly and knowledgeable employees who not only know their cheeses, they let you taste them before you decide. Love pizza...? How about sprouted grain crust, raw sauce, raw milk cheese, raw veggies? It can be done!

While the thought of raw meat may not appeal to you, it is still an option on a raw food lifestyle. I eat marinated raw salmon called gravlax, found at most markets where they stock the smoked salmon. I may take two of the four slices and match it with grapes and raw milk cheese, or put small pieces on sprouted crackers or my own homemade crackers for lunch, or chop all four slices into a salad for dinner (see the Recipes Section).

Start slowly, if you are still unsure of eating entirely raw. Begin with a raw lunch and raw side dishes at supper. Add raw food slowly into your diet, if that is the best way for you. Just the act of being conscious of what you are eating and how it is prepared is going to make a huge impact on you.

Or, do as I did and jump in with both feet, going raw completely from the start. I cannot begin to describe how good I feel when I eat this way, versus how awful I feel eating a very processed diet. Either way, you're going to benefit from the changes you make.

Did you know that there are sprouted breads and crackers? I didn't, when I started this journey. But, there are and they are available in the freezer section of your health food store or local market. Major food chains are beginning to carry more and more of these healthier alternatives.

Dehydrated rather than baked (which is simply dehydrating at high temperatures and altering the chemical makeup of the ingredients), they offer all of the benefits of raw sprouted grains, with none of the processed flour and gluten of baked bread products.

Better yet, if you have a dehydrator, make your own crackers, cookies, and fruit leathers and save a ton of money while making the flavor combinations you prefer. And, I confess, I truly prefer my own homemade dehydrated items to the store-bought variety.

So, I pile organically-grown raw tomatoes, cucumbers, bell peppers, baby spinach, and sprouts on my sprouted crackers. Sometimes, I add a bit of raw milk cheese, some marinated salmon, or a bit of raw hummus to vary my meals. How about a sprouted tortilla, filled with fresh delicious veggies tossed in homemade dressing? Or a spinach, kale, pine nut puree, inside folded lavash, with sweet, hot pepper jelly on top? I love that, in particular, for breakfast, as it really jump-starts my system.

I have scoured books and the Internet for recipes, along with making up my own, to add to my enjoyment of my meals. Pinterest.com did not exist when I started eating this way, but I love surfing the site and pinning great recipes to try. Raw is not just all-salad, all the time. I've included some recipes in the back of this book, to get you started. And there are a lot of places on the internet to find more.

I make raw salsa and raw hummus, both from organic ingredients, along with dehydrated tortilla chips. I learned to make raw nut milk, which my daughter drinks by the glassful. I fashion my own cereal from rolled oats, organic raisins, raw germinated almonds and seeds, cinnamon, and raw honey. Add a splash of raw nut milk and I had a healthy filling cereal.

When I want cooked salmon, I cook it by

dry grilling it with dill and lemon slices or I make a glaze of raw honey, miso paste, and sesame oil. You can just add coconut oil to your pan and cook it that way, for an amazing caramelized coating to the fish.

If I want steak, I buy a small really good cut and pair it with a large, raw salad that includes sprouted nuts and seeds and dried fruit. I do eat pasta, tossed with raw diced vegetables, olive oil, and spices (or fresh-squeezed lemon juice and basil), although I now prefer the raw alternative. Not every day but, now and then, I include a variety of foods in my diet.

This is the point where I admit that, when I went into remission, I let myself go off this healthy meal regimen. Here I am, ten years later, back to eating the way I should have all along. I grew extremely ill from an impacted gall bladder, gaining back a lot of weight as a result. In just three months after my surgery, however, I lost nearly fifty pounds, just by changing back to eating this way.

When I eat a raw, savory breakfast, I can feel the difference in my morning. My favorite is to make a puree of baby spinach, kale, pine nuts, a little olive oil and a pinch of salt. I slather the mixture between two very thin pieces of lavash and top with a very small portion of sweet, hot pepper jelly. I can feel this jumpstart my metabolism, and I never get that feeling of my blood sugar 'bottoming out' later in the morning, the way I do with sugary breakfast choices.

The most important thing to take away from this is to make healthier choices more often than not. To eat mindfully, away from television and cell phones, and focus on eating slowly, carefully, and on the people you're with. And, when you choose something that is less than good for you, eat it, enjoy it, and then go back to eating healthy. Don't beat yourself up for that meal. Look at the big picture and don't give up just because of a few bites of pizza.

A word of advice: if you work toward healthier eating and start to eliminate processed, high-salt and high-sugar foods, you may notice a few things happening. You may begin to get headaches, for example. You may also feel your food has no taste. And, you may start having very strong cravings for those very things you're trying to eliminate.

If this happens, you are probably detoxing. Your brain becomes addicted to processed food, sodas (both regular and diet), salt, and sugar, and you're going to have to experience some withdrawals if you ate a lot of that kind of food. These foods stimulate the pleasure center of the brain and your brain likes that... a lot. In addition, your taste buds have to adjust to the changes you're making.

You may also experience some bad breath, stronger-than-usual-smelling sweat, more frequent bowel movements, and other detoxing symptoms. These won't last long and they are a sign that your body is clearing itself out.

If you fall off the nutrition wagon, just climb back on. Don't beat yourself up or decide that you've lost all the ground you've gained. Just start again, where you left off. After about three months, in my experience, your tastes will change, and you'll really start to enjoy the healthier food. You are worth that investment of time and so is your well-being.

Mindful Eating

Mindful eating is an extension of both meditation and eating well. It focuses your attention on what you're eating and why you're eating it.

First, examine why you are reaching for a particular food. Emotional eating is a huge contributor to illness and weight gain. If you are seeking comfort from food, you may want to examine the deeper issues you're facing. I've been at the bottom of an empty flavored-tortilla chip bag and know that happens because I'm unhappy. It's worth taking a look.

When you do eat, be present. Do not watch television or surf the internet on your phone. This is not just a recommendation for the family meals of yore, though those are certainly something missing in our modern world. It's about paying attention to your food. At the very least, it should take as long to eat a meal as it does to prepare it.

Take your time in preparing your meal. Consider what to make and how the preparation can enhance the flavor and nutrition of each food. Balance your intake of protein, fat, sodium, and more. Try new flavor combinations. Experiment with new ingredients that will offer more energy, better healing, enhanced mood, and other benefits. Work with what's in season locally, as this will be the freshest and have the most to offer you nutrition-wise.

Portion your food, when it's ready, onto a pretty plate, taking stock of the colors and textures of what you're about to eat. Restaurants often offer a meal as beautiful as it is delicious, and there is no reason you cannot take a few extra moments to do the same.

Do this this with all you eat and drink, by the way. Use a favorite mug or a gorgeous vintage tea cup for your herbal, healing teas. Find a handmade bowl for soups and breakfast 'bowl' meals. Look for mismatched or lonely plates in a second-hand shop or treat yourself to one stunning bone china plate for your other meal choices Make it pretty, make it meaningful, and eat it mindfully.

When everything is ready, take a moment to be thankful. Whether you say a grace or simply focus on your gratitude for what you are about to eat, take a deep breath and breathe in gratitude, breathing out everything else.

Then, as you eat, notice each taste, each texture, each nuance of the food. Notice hot, warm, and cold. Notice spice, salt, and pepper. Chew consciously. Swallow and take a moment before taking the next bite. Be aware of the sun and rain and nutrients that went into the food. Be grateful for the hands that grew it, harvested it, and prepared it, even if they are yours, and the lives sacrificed. Savor every moment. And, then, mindfully, wash your dishes, dry them, and put them away for the next meal.

Gratitude is important here because it focuses us outside of our own bodies. It reminds us that we have more than we sometimes realize and that we can often get by on less than we want. And, by seeing the entire journey the food has taken to our plate, it connects us to the larger community in which we live. It is one thing to be grateful for food; it is another thing entirely to be grateful to every single being who contributed to your meal.

The more moments you take to slowly, mindfully eat your meals and snacks, the more slowly you will eat and the more you will benefit from your food. Even mindful sips of water, noticing how thirsty you are and then how satisfied, lead to more awareness of your body. Gratitude and pleasure can infuse every single meal and you deserve to let that happen.

Then, begin to carry that mindfulness over into each thing you do. Clean, mindfully. Bathe, mindfully. Converse, mindfully. Walk, mindfully. Create, mindfully. Interact with others, mindfully. We only have this one moment. Make the most of each one.

Remember, too, that it is often difficult to consider a lifetime to come that includes chronic illness. Instead, look to find joy in each moment. Nibble and savor your life in moments, and you'll find more joy than you ever imagined.

Meditation

"Live the actual moment. Only this actual moment is life. Don't be attached to the future. Don't worry about the things you have to do. Don't think about getting up or taking off to do anything. Don't think about 'departing'"
~ Thich Nhat Hahn, The Miracle of Mindfulness

In the fast-paced world in which we live, with our texting and insta-everything, the first response I get to the suggestion of meditation is that no one has the time. There is simply no time to set aside for sitting by oneself and meditating. I suspect it has more to do with feeling foolish and feeling selfish, for taking time for such frivolous pursuits, than an actual lack of time. The benefits, however, are well-documented and not just by me. I've listed several books in the back that explain the how's and why's of meditation, as well as the proven results.

The second objection is that people don't know how to meditate or, more to the point, don't know how to completely clear their minds. They have the idea that they have to sit on the floor, legs crossed, hands resting on knees, middle finger and thumbs forming perfect circles, and mind completely clear of any thoughts. The truth is you can meditate that way, but you can also meditate while walking or swimming. You can meditate while seated on a chair on your back porch or at your desk at work. Like anything else worth doing, the more you practice, the more easily you will achieve that which you seek.

I would add here that meditation can be practiced by those on any spiritual journey. Whether you call it meditation or prayer, it has more to do with opening your heart and quieting your mind than anything else.

I am not advocating one religion or one set of spiritual practices over another. I am advocating following your own spirituality to that place where you can be open and calm and at peace. For me, while prayer is speaking, meditation is listening.

To remind you, I felt no sensation in my

body at all but pain when I decided to take a different approach to my illness. Excruciating, burning, searing, mind-altering pain and nothing else. The touch of a friend's hand, the hugs of my children, the cool evening breeze, the soft bedcovers... everything hurt inside and out. Nothing had helped. No drugs. Not an intrathecal pump dumping pain medication directly into my spinal fluid. Nothing had helped me ease my pain at all.

I began slowly, by simply sitting outside in my backyard in the dark. I let my hands rest on my thighs as I breathed slowly in and out. I allowed sounds of human life to enter my thoughts and then pushed them aside. I allowed the sounds of animal life and the breeze in the trees to enter my thoughts, along with the scents of my garden, the smell of impending rain and the coolness or heat of the evening air. I focused on my breathing, in and out, slow and deep, feeling the air fill my lungs and then leave my body.

In the beginning, that is all I felt. It was peaceful. It was calming. It wasn't much else. Somewhere along the way, I began to focus on a particular tree or cloud pattern or star, allowing the image to fill my mind. I would close my eyes, keeping that image in my mind, and breathing slowly and deeply. It was when I could then clear my mind of that image that I found I could begin to transcend my pain.

What does that mean exactly? Here's how I described that first experience in my journal:

"Tonight was the full moon. It is a beautiful evening in my backyard, rare for NJ in July, as there was no humidity and the temperature was in the mid-70's. There was no breeze to exacerbate my pain. The air was slightly scented by some of my Knock-out roses as they begin to bloom again. Crickets sang loudly and lightning bugs seemed determined to gain my attention. Slightly cloudy skies meant only the brightest stars made it through the local ground light. Later, the moon will pass behind tall pines and oak trees.

Getting started was slow going. Though I have attempted meditation indoors and had some success, it has only been for calming or focus before studying. I have never reached past my pain on any attempt to meditate. Breathing deeply causes additional pain so I have to work up to it slowly. My neighbor's motion-detector lights were triggered by their dog at one point and a siren also deterred my first attempts to focus. Still, I calmed and began again. This night was a jewel that I was not going to pass up.

Finally, I found my center. I focused on the dark trees in the moon's impending path. Blacker than a black sky, the longer I looked at them, I began to see a faint glow in them, a shifting of energy around them. Then, I closed my eyes, holding the image of those trees in my mind.

Using the trees, I imagined my feet in the soft warm earth of summer. This is a very difficult step for me, as I am disconnected from the ground, my feet on the footrest of my wheelchair. I tried to remember the feeling of my feet in the grass and the dirt, to get beyond my chair. This time, I succeeded in feeling the warmth and the dirt between my toes. My feet became the roots, reaching further down into the earth, solid and sure.

Next, I pictured my legs, straight and strong, rather than withered and heavy. Rising tall from the roots, my hunched middle became the straight trunk and my weak arms joined the thick branches, outstretched toward the sky. On one side was night, dark, black, cool, and silver. On the other was day, bright and blue and warm. My branches embraced both, reached for both. My head was warm from the sunshine, my face cool from the moon. There was no pain, only joy. For the first time in more than eight years, I was in no pain and I was not in my weighted and useless body.

Then, suddenly, my dog barked and I fell back into place. I remember that very sensation of being out of myself and falling back, snapping back into place. The pain *engulfed me once more. I was unaware of crying until I leaned forward with my face in my hands, feeling rather worn out. It was not sorrow that caused my tears but that tiny glimpse of possibility. Instead of being angry or sad, I was thrilled and overjoyed. Even as I was exhausted, I was elated.*

As I write this, I am crying because it is there and I found it. There is a place outside of this pain that no drug or other intervention has eased to any degree. There is a place beyond the physical, where bodies no longer matter. I am still here inside all this pain and illness, and I found that 'me' tonight.

There is a particular piece of Celtic art that I have always loved. The Tree of Life has always called to me. What I felt tonight was me inside that Tree. I was the Tree. Well, whole, and strong, the Tree lives in me."

I felt compelled to draw out what I saw in those moments. The act of doing so kept me in that place of peace and connection, and it sparked my desire to create a form of healing art for myself (more on that in another chapter).

After I drew out that experience in colored pencils, I began to focus on the drawing when I meditated. It was easier, once I had succeeded, to find that place of peace and wholeness again. Now, I need only picture that image in my mind to go there again.

I continued my meditation exercises, sometimes journeying into the woods behind my home to reconnect with the Earth. It is easier to leave the world of humans behind there, feeling a part of some ancient past as the creek flows by. I have meditated under the full moon and felt its power and pull. I have encountered questions and answers in my meditations. I have found a peace there unequaled in my everyday life.

As you begin to meditate and find yourself succeeding, be sure to have a bite to eat and a sip of cool water when you finish. Place your feet firmly on the ground, your hands too if possible, to ground yourself when you finish. This is an important step and, if you are interrupted during your meditation, crucial to re-orienting yourself back to the present moment. Failing to ground yourself can lead to feeling lost and confused following any meditation work.

Do not feel you must clear your mind completely, become a 'blank slate' and sit in a lotus position to meditate. If clearing your mind seems impossible, you will find it impossible and give up before you ever succeed. You may find visualization (see below) works as a doorway to meditation for you instead. Remember, when something seems impossible, it will be. Thoughts become things. Find a way through, around, or over the closed door. Don't give up.

If you can't clear your thoughts, instead assign them to something and let them go. See them as leaves floating on a stream. See them, acknowledge them, let them flow away, and re-center. I've even put some more persistent thoughts into imaginary boxes, labeled them, and put them on imaginary shelves.

If you still have trouble meditating, seek out an experienced guide, someone who can help with guided meditation to get you started. There are plenty of books available with guided imagery and meditations as well. Check your local library or bookstore for suggested titles. Check online for CDs or downloadable guided meditations. I've listed a few at the end of the book to get you started.

Visualization

Visualization is a bit different. It is picturing the desired result in your mind in order to achieve that result. It is seeing yourself as well, for example, in a very specific way. For me, it was seeing myself walking. Seeing my children hug me without pain. Seeing my brain with no brain lesions. It is sometimes difficult for people to begin visualization, something we are not taught to do in our society.

Let me give you an example of visualization. What I want you to do is NOT to picture your bedroom. Do not see your bed, the color of the walls, or the flooring beneath your feet. Don't think of your comfortable pillow or the photograph by your bed.

Now, what happened? You pictured your bedroom. And, that is visualization!

Now, try closing your eyes and picturing an apple. See the color of the skin. Is it one solid color or does it change from green to red? Is the skin shiny or matte? Is it cool to the touch or warm from the sun? Are there any bruises or blemishes on the skin? Can you smell the scent of the apple? Can you see yourself cutting it open? Can you picture the juicy flesh inside, the sweet apple smell, the dark brown seeds? This is visualization.

Next, imagine yourself without whatever illness and symptoms you have. See yourself whole and strong and healthy. See yourself symptom-free. If you're in a wheelchair or use a cane, see yourself walking freely and steadily. Picture this over and over in your mind. See it. Believe it. Make it your daily mantra. Thank the Spirit that this is who you are inside and see it manifested on the outside.

If you've had trouble meditating, try seeing a garden in your mind. Plant it. Create it. Furnish it. Fence it with a little gate and arbor covered in morning glories. Is there a stream that runs through it? A large tree that shades you on hot days? A hammock or comfortable chair… or do you prefer to sit on the cool grass?

Create the garden of healing in your mind and go there whenever you need to retreat and regroup. Speak to Spirit there. Ask your questions and open your heart to receive the answers. Let your garden become your refuge from your illness and any other chaos in your life. You will reap what you sow in this garden and you will benefit greatly from your visits there.

Get moving

"Health is the vital principal of bliss, and exercise, and health." ~ James Thomson ~

Always consult your physician before beginning any exercise program.

Yes, exercise! Because as you begin to move, you will see other changes in yourself. Exercise increases endorphins, which in turn improve mood. Exercise can also improve sleep patterns, with sleep being vital to maintaining and even improving health. Just getting up and walking again saw me losing two clothing sizes in as many months. The same can be true for you, just be increasing the amount you move and exercise.

You can start by beginning to strengthen long unused muscles and tighten up areas, especially where weight loss takes place. Exercise will stimulate you and increase your appetite. You will eat more healthy food and drink more water and feel so much better overall. Exercise will stimulate your heart to pump more efficiently as well. You will look better and feel better about yourself. Exercise is a win-win situation.

You do not, however, need to immediately go out and join an expensive gym or club or purchase any equipment. Any results you want to achieve can be obtained by learning to listen to your body and to understand what you need. The same is true for exercise. No one knows better what you can do and what motivates you.

Remember to wear lose clothing and drink plenty of water while exercising. Choose those times of day you feel your best and the types of exercise you enjoy. Have an alternate option, in case weather affects your ability to exercise as you normally would (a yoga video for days you can't walk due to inclement weather, for example).

Keep your exercise in line with your level of commitment to it. If you have to drive somewhere, you probably won't go. If you have to drag out equipment, you probably won't do that either. Your exercise should fit into your life the way your new meals do. It should simply flow out of those things you enjoy doing. Then, it will become second-nature to you.

Walking is always a good choice for exercise. It gets you outside, in the fresh air, sunshine and the world around you. It's easy and it's free. It's low impact but high benefit. A good walk around the block, with good supportive shoes, is a great way to get out and get moving. Or find a local park that offers a path for walking. A walking buddy helps keep you motivated while keeping you company. A walking stick gives you confidence and support.

Personally, I found that having a group to walk with is a great approach. If more than one person is interested in walking once or twice a week, at least someone will be there with you, and probably more than one. You can talk while you walk, which keeps your mind off the exercise. And they will motivate you, encourage you, and cheer you on.

Don't forget to stretch a bit first, particularly your calves, before you begin your walk. I simply lean my hands on the wall, stretch my feet out as far behind me as I can while keeping them flat and the stretch each one several times before I begin to walk. Keep your pace just brisk enough to get your pulse up but not so much that you overtax yourself right away. Don't worry about how far you've walked or how many steps or how many minutes. Just walk until you feel you've pushed yourself a bit and gotten your heart rate up. If you do this several times a week, you'll see that you can go further and longer. And, if you do it this way, you'll be free to notice the changing of the seasons and the beauty around you as well.

Walking meditation is a great way to combine exercise with relaxation. No, that's not an oxymoron. Be mindful of each step you take, each breath in, and each one out. Be aware of your heart rate, the perspiration on your forehead, and the breeze that cools it. Clear away today's cares and tomorrow's worries to be in the moment of walking.

Feel your body push through, feel the muscles work and stretch, recognize when you feel fatigue, enjoy the way a drink of water refreshes you and moistens your throat. And, enjoy your arrival back home, to the sanctuary you may feel there.

Swimming and water work

Another ideal form of exercise is swimming. If you don't own a pool, you can usually join a local YMCA or other club to gain access to a pool. Many such facilities offer lifts if you need one. And, those places usually offer some classes for water exercises. If you own a pool or have access to one, try walking in the water around the perimeter of the pool, your hands moving back and forth as you normally would when walking, using the resistance to gain strength. This works arms and legs. Walk several laps in one direction and then turn and walk against the 'current' you've created. This adds additional resistance. I always stretch before doing this, as I do for walking, by leaning my hands on the side of the pool and stretching my calves and arms.

Swim laps of breaststroke, sidestroke and crawl, hold the side and kick against the water and do 'scissors' with your legs, walk around the perimeter… any form of exercise in a pool offers resistance and low impact. Swimming laps raises your heart rate as well. This is an excellent form of overall exercise if you are extremely overweight because the water adds buoyancy and, from personal experience, allows you to do far more than you can on dry land.

Other methods

There is another way to exercise that is very easy to fit into your schedule. Isometric exercises can be done anywhere, anytime. Any muscle can be tightened and released, as a form of low-impact exercise. This can be done unobtrusively while waiting at red lights, watching television, reading a book, working at your desk, anywhere, anytime. Simple, easy and very, very effective. Even in a wheelchair, isometric exercises can strengthen and tone muscle.

While at work, watching television or surfing the internet, lean back in your chair and tighten and release your stomach muscles. Do this over and over again, several sets a day to tone your abdomen. Hold your stomach in as you walk or swim, too. In bed, lay flat and tighten and release your buttocks, while holding your stomach in. This tightens and tones your backside and upper thighs. Tightening stomach muscles ultimately helps strengthen your back. Flex and straighten your feet, to strengthen ankles and calves and avoid 'drop foot'.

When you feel ready for more, don't rush out to the store and spend lots of money on special weights and equipment. A simple set of weights can be fashioned from two soup cans and a pair of socks. Drop one can in each sock, tie them at the top, and drape over ankles for weighted leg lifts and knee exercises and hold in your hand for arm curls. As you get stronger, use bigger cans.

A large ball from the market is cheaper than an 'exercise ball' but can work the same way for stomach crunches. I use an abdominal 'chair' to get me started, as it keeps my sciatica from sidelining my exercise time.

Heavy books can be lifted at arms' length to add weight to your efforts. Ride a bike.

Garden. Play catch with your kids or volleyball in the pool with them. Take lessons in horseback riding and connect with the power and beauty of the horse while you exercise (there are places that offer ramps to gain access to riding on horseback).

Do those things you love and push yourself a little while doing them. These things cost nothing but the long-term benefits are well-worth the effort. As always, stretch before and after exercising and drink plenty of water.

Libraries are a good source for exercise videos and DVD's. You can get beginner's level yoga, aerobics, Tai Chi and more... whatever appeals to you. Borrowing these before you purchase them allows you to try different types of exercise before you invest in something. Mail-order DVD services offer titles to try, and the MS Society offers videos as well. With any of these, you can work out in the privacy of your own home and at your own pace. Again, stretch before working out and after you finish, wear lose clothing, and drink plenty of fresh filtered water to keep you hydrated.

If you feel you need an instructor and a class to motivate you, check out the local support organization for your condition. They sometimes offer free or low-cost classes in yoga and other forms of exercise. Your local YMCA or church may also offer low-cost classes.

A note about drinking while exercising. Sports drinks contain sodium, artificial sweeteners, and other ingredients. Many bottled drinks, even some flavored 'waters', contain artificial sweeteners. Juices can also contain added sugars and high-fructose syrups. Your best bet is good, old-fashioned filtered pure water. In addition to re-hydrating your body and cleansing your system, water will also hydrate your skin.

If you still feel the need to flavor your water, infuse it with fresh organic herbs, fruit, and even cucumber. You'll gain the benefits and flavors without also adding unnecessary sugars and calories.

You'll never regret the benefits of drinking fresh water.

Flower pots

No, there isn't a mistake in the editing of the book. Yes, this section is really entitled 'flower pots'. Why? Because sometimes you need to express your feelings to get them out of your body. Anger, frustration, and stress take a terrible physical toll on us, if we don't express them and get them out.

One incredibly helpful piece of advice I received from a counselor is to throw flowerpots. First, find old, chipped terracotta flowerpots or even buy really cheap ones on sale. Old china works well too. You need something that will really smash well and give you a very satisfactory sound along with it.

Next, find a safe place, preferably with a vertical wall. Set a timer for two minutes (I'll come back to this) and throw the flowerpots as hard as you can against that wall, until the timer goes off. Rant, rail, vent, scream, wallow, and of course, throw those flowerpots. When the timer goes off, you have to stop. Stop throwing and stop wallowing.

The reason for the timer is simple. You have a set amount of time to get everything out of your system, but you won't get stuck in those feelings. You feel everything, own those feelings, but get them out, all at the same time.

After you've done this once or twice, or twenty times for those of us who are more stubborn, you won't actually need to throw pots any longer. Remember that visualization idea earlier? It works here too. Set the timer, visualize smashing the pots, and get those feelings out. Still works... but there are less pieces to pick up afterward.

Cry when you need to

There are so many people who won't cry. Whether they feel it makes them look weak or they fear letting go and not being able to stop, crying is seen as something to avoid. It actually is something that is important to your health and wellbeing. Crying relieves stress and lowers blood pressure. It even removes toxins from your system.

Ever feel like you need to cry but forced yourself not to? Ever get a headache from doing that? The exact opposite will happen if you just let the tears flow.

Again, you don't want to get stuck in the sadness but, the truth is, that is more likely to happen if you don't allow yourself to cry, than if you do. Just acknowledge the pain and sadness, cry it out, and move on.

Rest

Notice that I didn't say 'sleep'. There were months and months of me not being able to sleep, during my second relapse. Sleep was something that was just not going to happen with any regularity. So, I learned to rest.

Tossing and turning in bed for hours does not accomplish anything but frustration and, possibly, pulled muscles. So, at that point, it is better to get out of bed. However, you should not do anything stimulating. You should do something 'restful'. This will differ from person to person. For you, it may be reading. For me, it was writing.

I spent hours, often all night, writing. I went to a place writers call 'the flow' and wrote the stories I found there. The sun would rise, the alarm would go off, and I felt as refreshed as I did if I had slept through the night. When I could, I would nap. But writing became my rest.

You have to learn what your body needs and do that. You have to take time to sleep, if possible, and to rest, most assuredly. Quiet, dark, peaceful rest is possible, but you have to find the best way to obtain that for yourself.

Soft instrumental music, nature sounds, white noise, dim or dark, comfortable rest, for short periods of time may be all you can obtain at times. Be aware of what temperature is best for you, either too warm or too cool and you won't be able to relax. Soft sheets, cooling pillows, loose clothing... all these can contribute to a more restful experience.

Float in a pool to relax and cool off, meditate, curl up with an old movie or a great book. Your body needs sleep and rest to recover. Hopefully, rest will ease you into the sleep you so desperately need. Take it when it comes and consider it an obligation to yourself. Part of your self-care.

I used to fight taking naps, because I knew sleeping through the night to be the best thing for my body. If you're not sleeping through the night, however, naps are a good option. And, let's face it, as adults, stealing a nap here and there can be a delicious treat if we allow ourselves to grab it. Like chocolate and other things, naps and sleep are definitely good for the body and the soul.

Inner Work

"The space you carve out of your life is the place where magic will happen, the place where you will grow, be healed, and changed." ~Michael Samuels, MD, and Linda Rockwood Lane, Ph.D., Creative Healing~

Many, many, many of us carry within us inner wounds that also need healing. I am not speaking here of physical wounds. I am referring to spiritual, emotional, and psychological wounds. And, I am referring to soul loss.

Any time we experience trauma, our souls splinter off to protect us. Sometimes, those splinters filter back into us. But, other times, they stay separate and we lose them or surrender them to someone else. This is soul loss. Over the course of a lifetime, depending on the number and kinds of traumas we face, we can lose tiny bits or large pieces of ourselves. And, those losses differ from person to person.

Western medicine generally attempts to

address physical symptoms when a person experiences physical illness, or to recreate chemical balance when someone has mental instabilities, with medications. You have pain, you take a pain killer. If you've been abused, you go into therapy or counseling to understand what and why.

However, many illnesses are the direct result of unaddressed soul loss. They are real illnesses, but they go much deeper than our skin and our muscles. Only when the splintered-off bits of our souls are returned to us do we truly become whole. And, this is the difference between being well and being whole. This is the difference between healing and curing. My illness is all too real, I assure you, but it goes much deeper than lesions in my brain. I am not only seeking physical healing. I have experienced the healing of my soul.

I will not go into details of the traumas I have suffered. That I suffered at the hands of others is what matters. That I surrendered bits of myself contributed to my soul loss. That others took my power, or that I gave it away in order to 'keep the peace' and to maintain the status quo. I have been a card-carrying enabler and I have the 'flaming codependent' tee shirt.

My weight ballooned as my self-esteem and self-image diminished. I endured physical, emotional, and psychological abuse and, being the enabler and co-dependent that I am, I I didn't even realize what was happening. Each surrender of myself resulted in a small bit of my soul leaving me. Thread by thread, the unraveling of my soul began.

In addition, I had to stay where I was. You may have asked yourself why a victim of abuse stays? Here's one reason: if I had left, when I was so very sick, I would not have been given custody of my children. I had to stay, for them. Once full-blown, complete remission set in, the tables were turned and I was able to literally stand up and say 'no more'. That renewed physical strength also opened the door to digging deeper.

As a result, part of my journey toward wholeness involved inner work. Deep, intense meditations took me inward to see where the holes were in my soul and inner journeys sent me looking for those missing pieces. This is difficult work and should be undertaken only when you are fully prepared for it. There are psychologists, clergy, and trained shamans who assist in soul retrieval and a myriad of books explaining how and why this is necessary. I have listed some of my favorites at the end of this book. Difficult work, yes, but, it is necessary.

This is not to say that soul retrieval is the be all or end all, just as one pill doesn't cure every illness. I see it as one of the many tools we need to employ in order to become truly well and whole. Used in conjunction with a raw, organic regimen, meditation, visualization, and psychological counseling, and, yes, Western medicine, the other tools in your toolbox, soul retrieval is extremely beneficial to our overall well-being.

I can give an example here of the physical manifestation of imbalance in the soul. I experienced migraine headaches throughout my life, though in the beginning they were rare. Interestingly, the frequency and severity of my migraines increased the further I went in counseling and soul work. Their onset devolved to full-blown migraines much more quickly. I reached the point of weekly migraines, even as I began to heal psychologically from my counseling. It took me months to see the connection.

When there was soul work to be done, but day-to-day life interfered with the work, I would end up with a migraine. I manifested physical pain from unresolved soul loss. Once I realized the connection, and responded to that work immediately as it arose, my headaches disappeared.

Another way to look at this comes from the very illness I live with. One day, medical science will discover a cure for what I have. Some drug or therapy will halt the symptoms from continuing and there will be no new cases. But, is that the end of it? What about all those physical and cognitive losses we have suffered at the hands of the monster? Will the cure reverse them or will there be more work to be done? Soul work is the 'more' that we need to do to heal our souls.

Soul retrieval is one more step toward balance and wholeness. The trauma of major illness, death, financial devastation, abuse, terror, and other stressors in our lives will not cease while we live and breathe. But, knowing that they can rob us of our soul allows us to address those losses before or as they occur, so that we do not have to struggle to survive without that which makes us who we are.

I read books to learn more about how to identify soul loss and how to renew my soul. I also did my own meditations, to visit those wounded places within myself and bring light and healing to them. This is neither simple nor easy, as you must go to the very darkness most of us shun and fear. Just remember, without the darkness and chaos of the cocoon, there would be no butterfly.

Again, this process can be guided by your own spiritual beliefs and within any religion. It is important that it is true to who you are, for it to be effective.

Picture an old house, dilapidated and abandoned. Hanging from a broken, crooked window is the remnant of what was once a lace curtain. Now, it hangs limp and dingy, shredded and filled with gaping holes, only moving slightly in a chilled breeze. It neither protects from outside storms nor enhances the space within. You have a sense that it once was something special and you long to know what it may have looked like before it was left to decay.

Now, picture a magnificent home, not overly large or opulent, but substantial and welcoming and cozy, both inside and out. In a lovely window made up of straight lines and sparkling glass is stunning piece of lace, unique and intricate. It is clearly a vintage curtain, though there are no stains or yellowing. It just speaks of material handmade with love and care and of caretaking from the heart, of valuing that which is both delicate and strong.

Both images are mine, both are my soul. The first image is my soul for many decades, abandoned and shredded by illness, pain, and abuse. The missing pieces both lost and hidden away, and it seemed it could never be repaired, let alone be what it once was.

Souls are old, connected to the Universe, born of the stars. Living, choices (both our own and those of others), illness, and pain can change and even wreak havoc on our souls. We lose pieces. We hide others away to keep them safe from further harm, and we hide with them. We create a different persona, a reflection of that altered soul.

The second image is also my soul when I was a child, until the age of four. And, it is my soul now. I have found a way to renew and reclaim, to re-weave and re-stitch, to lighten and whiten and brighten. I have retrieved that which was lost and I have unearthed that which was hidden.

I now am myself, and all that means. I am unedited, unapologetic, and unabashed. I am flawed and fabulous, brazen and beautiful. I still have a lot of work to do, a lot of things to accomplish, and a lot of love to give this world.

While I love fully and completely, and give my gifts to all I can, I will never again relinquish bits of my soul for any reason. I can do better, I can do more, I can offer more, if I am true to myself, than I ever could when I lived in a way that was inauthentic and incongruent.

Then sings my soul, making a joyful noise, and it is my song that I sing. Mend your spirit, repair your soul, and sing your own unique song. The world needs your song as much as you do.

Faith

Faith has always been a part of my life. I was blessed with two parents who 'walked their talk' and whose strong faith influenced my own. I was also blessed with one clergyman in particular, who honestly told me that he would not even begin to attempt to address the 'why' of the horrific pain I lived with. He didn't sugarcoat it or tell me it was a test of my strength. He didn't compare me to Job or tell me 'God had brought me to it'. He empathized with me. He suffered with me. And he made tangible, measurable efforts to ease what my family faced as a result of my illness.

Faith is believing in that which we cannot see and cannot feel. It's believing in the impossible when nothing else seems possible. It's knowing, without rhyme or reason, that we will make it through whatever we face and that we are never facing it alone.

If friends and loved ones are lifelines, faith is an anchor.

Faith leads to hope and hope leads to an unchained spirit. Knowing that you can do more than your body wants you to believe involves a great deal of faith. Faith in doctors and faith in our loved ones, to do what is best for us and to be there for us when we need them most. Faith, that we are made of strong stuff. Faith, in all that we can still do. Faith, that there is God and Spirit and a Universe that all conspired to create us. Faith puts things into perspective and gives our lives purpose.

What is important is that you know what it is you believe, that you have the faith to take the journey, that prayers of gratitude are part of your daily regimen no matter what happens, that you pack all the tools you will need, and that you follow that to an unchained spirit.

Friends – Anchors, lifelines, and spoons

With faith as your anchor, friends are your lifeline. Family and friends who see you within the illness and who are there for you through anything (and everything) keep you from going down the third time. Hang on tight to, and appreciate, true friends and true love. It doesn't matter how many there are; it matters who they are for you.

Lifelines

As the heading implies, we need lifelines when we live with chronic illness. People we can count, truly count on, keep us grounded and tethered so we are not adrift and feeling all alone. So, who can we count on?

First, look for friends who are true lifelines when you need them most. They are there first. They will do anything. They truly understand, and they will also back off without being offended when asked. They are the ones who simply pick up where you left off, when there has been time apart, and they are those who will come looking for you when you've been quiet too long.

You always hear that you find out who your true friends are in a crisis, and I have found that to be true. My most recent test saw every single one of my friends stepping up to help, support, love, and listen. I learned that I had found my true community, my true Tribe, where I am right now. It was not always that way.

There was a day when I learned that those I had counted as friends were not. A crisis of epic proportions tested their professed friendship and found it lacking, in very big ways. I was left standing on a front lawn, waiting for the police to arrive, rather than allowed into the safety of a neighbor's home. I was also berated for calling the police in the first place by those whom I previously had thought cared about my children and me.

Yet, at the same time, people I had thought were acquaintances, some people I barely knew, stepped forward to offer love and safety to me and to my children. A neighbor I had never met gave me a key to her house, as a safe haven for my children. I can tell you that three true friends beat twenty not-quite friends in any scenario.

You've heard that saying 'any port in a storm'? Well, I'm going to tell you to forget that one. Any port in a storm will most certainly NOT do. Better to brave the storm on your own for a while longer, than to take on someone toxic or someone downright dangerous. And there are those who appear as friends who are there for rather more nefarious reasons. So, how to weed out your true friends?

What do they ask of you and what do they offer? Take a step back and 'gut test' the relationship. Are you happy to see them or do you feel nervous? Are you walking on eggshells or relaxed and happy when you're together? Do they talk about others, like gossip or criticism and, if so, could they be doing the same about you? Do they expect more than you are able or willing to give or do you feel blessed by having them in your life? It's really not the quantity of friends that matters. It's the quality of the friendship.

Borrowing spoons

"Shouldn't you, I don't know, save up the good for the less-than-good days?" – Sam, Love in the Middle. If only we could…

By now, you may have heard of The Spoon Theory by Christine Miserandino. If not, look it up. It gives you the words to explain what it's like to have MS or Lupus or some other chronic illness to a healthy person. Not an easy task but one the spoon theory takes on well.

My reason for bringing it up here is not to reinvent the spoon. It's been done to perfection by Ms. Miserandino. What I want to talk about is borrowing spoons, not from the next day but from other people.

One of the most difficult things to learn, when faced with a chronic illness, is letting other people help you. I say this, knowing full well that even after three decades, I still struggle with this. My kids and friends will read the first line of this paragraph and give me the 'do what now?' look. I would have no trouble at all helping anyone, anytime they needed me. Letting them help me? That's where I have a problem.

Borrowing spoons might be easier for us to do if we could trade them. "I'll do this for you today, because I am able to. I'll borrow one of yours when I need it (and you're up to it)." The thing is, true friends want to help, feel a burning need to help, and might honestly be a little hurt if you don't let them help. They are at a loss as to what to do for you.

Seriously, why can't Sue do your laundry for you one day, other than your stubborn pride? If you need it done and are out of spoons, let her help! It makes her feel better. It gets your laundry done. Everyone wins.

When and if you do borrow a spoon or two, be patient when your helper does things differently than you do. Does it really matter if Bill folds the shirts differently than your usually fold them? Or if Kim puts the silverware in a different slot in the drawer. I know I feel better if my house is uncluttered and laundry is folded and put away. Your friend might feel the same. Why not trade off when you need to?

Relax, welcome the help, mute the correcting, and accept the spoon.

Intimacy, relationships, and illness

This is not a book that is going to tell you that everything will always be all right, and that life as you knew it before diagnosis will continue on as it always has. You are exactly the same person you were when you went to that appointment, but part of that definition of 'you' now includes a diagnosis of chronic illness. You may stay where you are, health-wise, indefinitely. You may have great days. You may have awful days. And that makes having relationships challenging. Let's get real here.

Relationships and intimacy can suffer in chronic illness, in ways that are difficult to put into words. He may be afraid to touch you, for fear of hurting you. She may be hesitating to approach being romantic, for fear you're not in the mood. Or she may feel so 'unsexy' that she projects an assumed lack of interest onto you. Medications play havoc with our taste, touch, breath, and bodily functions, and sometimes our sex drive. Incontinence makes us feel completely unsexy.

Information on this subject is often either very clinical or grossly oversimplified. There is only so much you can read about being sure you're clean, smell good, brush your teeth, and talk things through with your partner. The truth is, you may have to work together to redefine 'intimacy', just as you must now redefine 'normal'. It may, at some point, look very different than you're used to.

By the way, I'm all for smelling and looking your best, but you also need to think of ways to be close, in spite of your symptoms. When our bodies betray us, we may need to add to our bag of tricks to please and pleasure our partners and find what works for both of you.

The main thing is to touch, kiss, snuggle, spoon, and laugh together as much as possible. Make love all the time, by being loving and caring. Do all you can for one another. Do the things you love to do together on good days, and curl up together on bad days.

Chronic illness is a test for any relationship and a deal breaker for many. You don't have to be a statistic, though. You can be a force of two, in fighting and living well in spite of illness.

This is a difficult section to write because I do not want to scare you and because people usually don't want to talk about intimacy. I do want to prepare you, though. And I want others to know that, behind closed doors and forced smiles, relationships are falling apart. We say the words "in sickness and in health, for better and for worse" but do we mean them? Or do we mean, "as long as I don't have to carry the load virtually alone, because you are ill"?

I read posts on the internet all the time, heartbreaking and gut-wrenching posts about how the spouse who does not have MS "doesn't deserve this" and "didn't sign up for this". Well, of course, no one deserves this. But, hell, yes, he or she mostly certainly did sign up for it. They did when they said they loved us and made a commitment to us.

Would they expect such understanding, if they were the one being left for something they had no control over? What are we signing up for, exactly, when we make a commitment to someone, if not this very thing? Love is easy when life is easy, but love is truly worth it when life is challenging.

Yes, by all means, talk things through, especially intimacy. Talk about what you need and what your partner needs. Prepare for changes with things like lubricant, so that neither of you has to worry about pain. Say what hurts, say what feels good, say what you long for. And ask the same of your partner. Like anything that makes us uncomfortable, this might be difficult in the beginning. But, it's worth that to get to the good stuff.

Remember to talk about other things too. The illness cannot and should not be the main thing you both share. It should not be the focus of your life together. Remember what brought you two together in the first place and make sure you never lose sight of that.

You can also do things to feel better about yourself, even as you deal with your symptoms and their challenges. Let's say you have to wear incontinence underwear. Seriously not sexy, right? We really do need someone to design haute couture disposable underpants.

In the meantime, buy the sexiest bra you can afford. Or maybe lovely short silky nightgowns or camisoles. Buy funny or silky boxer shorts to put on over those disposables. Take the extra moment to feel good about yourself and put on something that feels good to you, to help you feel more relaxed and ready for your partner. You deserve sexy underwear as much as the next person. Treat yourself and fill that prescription.

Try scented or flavored oils for a couple's massage. Try being intimate in different places, that may be more conducive to being comfortable. Remember to snuggle, touch and talk before and afterward. Remember to snuggle, touch, and talk at other times too. Being close all the time can truly make a difference in feeling comfortable when you want to be even more intimate.

And please, laugh together! While an ill-timed 'toot' can threaten to break a mood, the ensuing laughter can bring you closer together and help you let go of your worry. Fears about stress incontinence during sex might be less of a worry if you fool around in the shower. Slip, slide, a little leak, and laugh about it... together. Age has some of these same effects on our bodies, so you're just getting a jump on learning how to handle all of that and be intimate at the same time.

Can't cook any longer? Ask a friend to prepare your partner's favorite meal for the two of you as a surprise (remember to trade spoons so you feel better about asking). Order take out from his favorite restaurant. Pick up her favorite candy every once in a while. Spend time in the garden together and surprise him with new plants or accessible tools if that's his passion. Drive to the beach to watch a sunset, with a picnic basket. Go to watch the fireworks.

Be a couple whenever possible. Be intimate in new, as well as tried-and-true ways. Even if your relationship wasn't tested by illness, it will be tested by other things through the years. Life happens to all of us. It won't feel like 'working at it' if you always consider the other person too.

When my father died very suddenly one morning, we all learned a very touching lesson in love and respect. For two years, because of her own physical challenges, my mother had been experiencing assisted living in her own home. Why didn't she know this? Because my father loved her so much, he wouldn't take away her car keys when he realized she should no longer be driving. Instead, he just happened to have an errand to run every single time she had to go out.

She hadn't done the laundry because, again, he just happened to have to go down into the basement at that moment, each time. She hadn't even put her own house key in the door lock because of the way he handled things. She never even realized it was happening. He treated her with love, respect, and kindness, the hallmark of their fifty-three-year marriage.

Ask any couple that has been together thirty years or more and you'll hear words like 'respect' and 'laughter'. If you each continue to focus on what makes the other person happy, you can still enjoy a committed, loving relationship that cannot be marred by illness or any other challenges you will face.

Making Lemonade

I am a big believer in making lemonade out of lemons, as cliché as that may sound. I am also someone who believes we should start as soon as the lemons present themselves. Often, we look for the silver linings of our challenges after the storm as passed. We assess the damage, evaluate what happened, why it happened, and what we learned from it. We hold onto the lemons until we have enough to make a full pitcher.

The thing is, we miss a lot by waiting. Gifts, lessons, and other serendipities may go unclaimed by waiting. I say, start picking those lemons from day one and squeeze 'em right away. Make lemonade by the glass, by the sip if you have to. And, while you're at it, dance a little in the rain of those storms.

Creative outlets

I do not believe that there is anything we

face that can keep us from being creative souls. I say this because I spent a very long time in a wheelchair, almost a decade and, yet, found creative outlets. I know a young woman who writes both fiction and non-fiction, paints and draws, and devours research on a regular basis, all using her mouth to perform these tasks because she is a paraplegic.

You might be saying, *well, sure they can do that but I can't*. Well, yes, you can. Degas did not stop creating when he began to lose his eyesight. He switched to clay, so that he could feel what he was creating.

If you already know where your creative talents lie, it's simply a matter of adapting to continue using them. Simple, in the sense of knowing where to start. Creativity does not lie in your hands or in your eyes, but in your brain, your heart, and your soul. Your unique talents are gifts you are meant to share with the world and you should continue sharing them, even when faced with physical challenges.

Why? Because you know what it means to tap into 'the flow' from where all art waits. You already know what it feels like to have hours spent drawing or writing or painting or sculpting feel like moments instead. You know what it feels like to get lost in the art, only to discover an amazing result when you 'wake'.

This is the very unchained spirit of which I write. This is the 'you' that is not trapped in a weighted or painful body. This is proof beyond measure that our souls reside outside of our troubled bodies and are not ill at all.

If you have not found your creative niche, there is no better time than when living with a chronic illness. For all of the reasons I've offered above, you can find a passion and pursue it. One of the only things I ever found to help me cope with the excruciating pain of my second relapse was writing.

When my children were little and they couldn't sleep, I used to tell them to make up stories to help them drift off. It always worked for them, so, when I couldn't sleep for the pain, I gave that a try myself. The stories became so entertaining that I began to write them down. At one point, I had more than seventy-five stories, some of which were complete novels.

In those long, dark hours of the night and the quiet days I was alone, my writing took me away from my situation and my pain. It wasn't that I did not feel the pain. It was simply a way to escape it for a time, to live within it and, I suppose, I lived within my stories. My body was stuck in a wheelchair, but my mind could go anywhere and everywhere.

It was a way to have a life, even if it was an imaginary one. As the pain continued to worsen, I continued to write my stories. I had no idea where the writing would ultimately take me and, honestly, I didn't care. To this day, I am still writing, honing my craft, and tapping into that all healing, all inspiring flow.

The beauty of creating something, anything, is that it takes you outside your own challenges and losses. You feel good about yourself. You feel good about what you make or bake or add to the world. It is a beautiful therapy for depression. And it gives you hope.

Because if you can create, you can live. You *are* living.

Art as Healing

I did not come to the realization of how to deal with my illness on my own. I felt alone. I thought it was only me. But, I have since learned to listen to the Stillness, to journey into the Dreamworld, and it was there that Spirit told me what to do. I am and will always be grateful for those silent conversations.

I knew I had done my first two carvings (The Greenman and my walking staff), thinking that I was manifesting hope to a tangible result. I had faith that, if I carved the walking stick, infusing it with my intentions, I would one day walk with it... and I did! I drew my drawing of my 'Unchained Spirit', the visible expression of what I had seen was truly possible. Looking back at those works, I see now what else resides in them. They were not just the hope I would become well. They were the means to that end.

The value of art in healing is incalculable. Art Therapy is an established mode of communicating one's inner pain, turmoil, and healing...its effectiveness proven time and time again. But, what happened to me was different. I was not communicating that which needed to be healed and having the symbols interpreted by a therapist. I was using the art itself as a means of being healed. I was creating that which could happen, that which was possible, with the assistance of Spirit. I was transforming my illness into wholeness, one work at a time. This is the power of art as healing. This is something altogether different.

Imagine playing with finger paints just for the sake of the play. Imagine pouring yourself into the pages of a novel or lines of poetry. Imagine sliding your hands into slippery clay and finding a precious pot or sculpture inside. Imagine examining a rainbow and then transferring those colors to a watercolor that reflects all the things you are feeling at once. Imagine actually dancing with joy or with sorrow when you feel those feelings.

Imagine raising your voice in song, your inner song, all alone in the middle of a deep, dark wood, or on a large rock with the crashing waves for accompaniment. Imagine communing with seeds as you plant them, or with plants as you purchase them, and creating a garden that ultimately heals the environment as much as it heals you.

It is not about whether the finished work is saleable or even if it speaks to anyone else (though it is my experience that it does... loudly). This is not about whether you have been born with talent or cannot draw a straight line with a ruler. It is about the work transcending the pain and healing the illness within.

Whether the pain is physical or emotional, whether the illness has treatments within modern Western medicine or defies all the doctors put together, art transcends all and heals the artist. Then, the artist can create in order to heal others and ultimately the Earth.

Art is transformative.
Art is expression.
Art is communication.
Art is healing.

Connecting with and creating art has been shown to positively impact those who are dealing with dementia, as well as those who are socially isolated or enduring ongoing illness. Creating art reduces anxiety and lessens depression, giving people a renewed sense of purpose, promoting self-discovery, and creating community.

And, so, another fascinating and exciting approach to healing can be found through art. Whether you are someone already familiar with creating personal art or someone who last created a finger-painting in kindergarten makes no difference. Healing with art works for anyone and everyone.

All you need to do is close your eyes and imagine what you'd like to do. Have you always admired watercolor paintings and wished you could do that? Have you secretly dreamed of writing the great American novel? Do you love to stare at paintings by the masters? Did you once enjoy playing with clay in grade school?

Maybe you were told by an unfeeling art teacher that you shouldn't come within a mile of pencil and paper. I was, in first grade. Boy, was she wrong! Because art is not in perfection. Art is in the intention. And, healing art has special intentions just for you.

What you do is first create, in any medium that speaks to you, art that speaks of your inner pain and turmoil. Draw it, sculpt it, define it in poetry... it doesn't matter as long as it's honest and comes from inside you. Then, create art of who you are, in your soul, well and whole. See it in your mind, visualize it, and then create it. Manifest it. Make it real. The art will help make it happen.

There is time for creating art in your life, if you see just how important this is. One half-hour a day, one pad of paper or one corner of the kitchen, and you're off and running. Dedicate that small space and small amount of time to becoming whole. You will never regret it.

This is where my writing began my journey toward healing. I was writing characters and situations that ultimately became part of my healing experience. My characters were voicing pain, abuse, and more that I never ventured to say out loud. They were in a safe place and could reveal the inner pain and scars that I could not. The catharsis that resulted opened the flood gates and released my inner artist.

Now, I cannot imagine a day in which I do not create something. Now, just the act of bringing something beautiful into being continues to heal me, and ultimately changes the world around me too. Find your inner artist and recreate yourself!

When you have a headache, do you take an aspirin? If you break your leg, do you allow the doctor to x-ray it and then cast it? Why is it different for a broken spirit or an aching soul?

Yet, if I said to you that you should set aside time every single day, even just a half hour, to find your inner artist and heal yourself, I'll bet you'd say you can't do that. You're too busy. Too many other demands have your attention. Or, you're a college student or a mom or single parent or adult caregiver, and you don't get a half hour to yourself.

Or you'll tell me you have no talent. You may once have marveled at the feel of clay in your hands or the shading of pastels on paper.

As a child, maybe you colored on the walls and got in trouble for it (I did). You may have yearned to try your hands at watercolor or the great American novel is still waiting inside you to be written. Your two left feet keep you from dancing. Your lack of formal training stills your song, and you could never create perfect works of art. Well, healing art is not about being perfect. It is, however, about being good enough.

All you need is intention. Create a space that is only yours. This could be a pad of paper, a lap top, a clear spot on the kitchen table, a bag of art supplies, a clear corner of your mind, a space in the yard for a new garden bed, or a desk all your own. It could even be *gasp* a room of your own.

Create that space with intention, the way you would prepare for any ritual. See the emptiness of the page or the screen or the silence as an invitation to create. Use aromatherapy to open your senses. Play music that opens your soul's ear. Have no expectations of what will happen or what the finished product will be. Such expectations actually inhibit. Be uninhibited. Color outside the lines. Think outside the box. In fact, toss out the box!

Close your eyes today and make a wish. Imagine a white fluffy dandelion, make a heart wish to find your inner artist, and then blow on the seeds. See them fly off in all directions, planting the seeds of intention in your heart and soul. Then, set aside one half hour, pick up the pen, the brush, the trowel, the guitar, the spoon, the clay, or whatever medium speaks loudest to your heart... and create.

Free the inner artist inside you and allow the art you create to heal you. Create art that speaks of your physical illness or your emotional turmoil. Create art that shows you healed of those very conditions. Free your Spirit of your chains and let your inner artist lay healing hands upon you. Let go of expectations and criticisms. Be generous with your Self. Let your soul speak through your healing hands and feet. Welcome the song that has been waiting to be sung and sing it with all your might.

Art is not in perfection.
It is in the intention.
This is healing at its finest.

My art continues to heal me and redefine me. It connects me to Spirit. But, I want to do more. I want to help others heal with my art. I want to heal the Earth and the world around me with my art. I want to make a difference and add to the beauty and balance of this world in which we live, by inspiring and encouraging others to create their own healing art. I want to offer back the tiniest portion of which I have been so abundantly blessed.

There is no "I can't" in healing art. There is

no "I'm not talented enough." Healing art is about what you've always wanted to try your hand at but were afraid to try. What you used to love to do but haven't done in forever. What made your heart race and your soul sing once upon a time... this is the art of your Spirit.

In Celtic spirituality, there is a belief in the opening up of the soul to enlightenment. It's called 'Imbas' and it is seen as the opening up of the top of one's head to allow Spirit to enter and enlighten. This is the perfect description of what it feels like to open your soul to creativity. And, when you do open that door to your own creativity, Spirit will push it wide open and bowl you over with it.

See your inner artist/healer as a very old music box. The case is dusty, the cylinder is tarnished, the springs tight and rusty, the song silenced. The box is locked and the key has been missing for a very long time. Yet, even so, there is a resonance surrounding it, as if the air around the box is vibrating with a song that has not yet been sung.

Healing art is the key that unlocks the song of the sacred spring of your soul. It oils the springs, brightens the cylinder, and turns the crank. It is there, waiting, whenever you are ready to begin... Let it open you up and speak for you.

There is a proverb that says, "The body heals with play. The mind heals with laughter. The spirit heals with joy." There are so many things that can rob us of that joy, though. When it comes to chronic illness, especially chronic pain, joy can seem an elusive will-o'-the-wisp, taunting us to follow and yet never quite 'get there'. That is why it's important, no, essential that you seek joy in your life on a daily basis.

I love two people who live within the unrelenting cloud of anxiety. At times, it is debilitating. Always, it is exhausting for them. They see all that could go wrong and perseverate on that. I try, as often as possible, to remind them that to face each day with anxiety takes a tremendous amount of courage and strength. They each look in a mirror and see a mouse. I look at them and see lions. You are no less a lion when you live every day with a chronic illness.

What do you see when you look in the mirror?

Is it all in how you spin it? Sometimes it is. You've heard 'fake it 'til you make it'? Long before someone coined that phrase, my mother used to tell me to wear red on days when I felt less than stellar. She said the color would brighten my face, along with lifting my mood. Sometimes, you need to wrap your soul in bright colors to achieve that same effect.

Perhaps your joy, your victory, for that day is taking a shower. Well, revel in the hot water, the feel and smell of the soap on your skin, the warming of tired, sore muscles. Perhaps you are so worn out, there is nothing you can accomplish. Then, sit back with headphones and listen to your favorite music. Just relax and be.

Sit outside and enjoy the sun on your head and the sound of the birds. There is an art to doing 'nothing' in this day and age, and it's one many of us have not practiced. Though I suffered terribly from sensory overload in the past, I still loved the loud, happy sounds of my children playing. I found joy in that.

I was asked once how it is that I wake up happy every day, by someone who truly had no idea such a thing was possible. How do I do it? I just do. First of all, I'm waking up. As Anne of Green Gables' beloved teacher would say, "today is a day with no mistakes in it." I can put my feet on the floor and stand. I can walk. I have a day of new choices and new possibilities ahead of me.

No matter what the day may bring, I have no reason not to be happy upon waking. I have no reason not to reflect on all that for which I am grateful at both the beginning and end of my day. How I view it is a choice.

Whatever has happened to me, or is even

happening right now, I have so much to be happy about. So many things to do; so many words to write. I have had to learn to find joy in each moment. Just as thoughts and behaviors that can drag us down can become habits, so too can finding joy and being happy.

You may have to search for joy. For many of us, especially when we live with chronic illness, it comes in fleeting moments, rather than in hours. Yet, it is an important element to living a full life, especially when living that life includes illness.

Build a community

This is so important. Do not just hide yourself away. And, do not just go on as if nothing is happening. You need to build a community around you, to share, support, and uplift one another.

This does not have be only people who share your chronic condition or serious illness, although people who do will be quick to understand when you need a sympathetic ear. This should be a group of people who know you, love you, and share interests with you of all kinds.

My Tribe, as I have come to call them, is comprised of hundreds of internet friends and an almost equal number of face-to-face friends. I have creative friends, writing friends, and friendships based on all kinds of interests I share with others. Having people there, in one way or another, means never having to be alone unless you choose to be alone.

It also means that you can be there for others, which takes you out of your own head. We sometimes get so used to going through the motions, just getting through the day, that our world shrinks to just that. A community keeps you feeling connected and allows the healthy give-and-take that beneficial relationships offer us. Find yours and fill that prescription.

Find your gifts

What are you good at doing? What is it that other people come to you for? What have you always dreamed of doing? What talent would you like to hone?

This is the best time to pursue your personal gifts. We all have them. We have all been blessed with them from the day we were born. You may have been discouraged from offering them to the world, but now is the time to dust them off and polish them up.

Why? Because now is the time for you to feel needed. Yes, you need to say 'no' when you are unable to step up. At the same time, you need to offer that gift back to the world, to keep you aware that you have a purpose, a reason for being here, even if you're battling some chronic illness. You are the hero on this quest, the one battling the monster, and you have inherent gifts that you can share with the rest of us.

Do you always make those around you laugh? That's a gift! Can you make beautiful art? Write beautiful stories? Those are gifts. Are you a talented and prolific baker? Yup, that's a gift. Are you the quintessential worker bee? Guess what? That's a gift!

This is so important, right now, because we can often lose our sense of self to illness. We spend a lot of time at the doctor's office, the lab, the pharmacy, where we become our patient ID or record number. We have to sort our pills and take our shots. We have to exercise and eat right. Everything seems geared toward the illness. Focusing on your gifts takes you out of the illness mode and puts you back into living.

Humor

You probably already know that I prefer to deal with my illness through humor. How? Because of the subtitle of this book. What I not-so-affectionately call my 'MS stupids' cause a lot of forgetfulness. I'd rather laugh at what life brings me than give up. After all, they say that laughing at a bully puts him in his place and there is no bigger bully than chronic illness.

There is a reason children focus a lot of attention on bathroom humor. Anything they are told is taboo becomes a source of amusement. We are no different as adults. Unless, that is, illness is involved. Then, we feel it is inappropriate and even hurtful to laugh.

Yet, laughter really is the best medicine. Look at Josh Blue, who has Cerebral Palsy, and Drew Lynch, who developed a severe stutter after an accident. Comedians like these gifted men allow us a chance to laugh with them and even to laugh at ourselves. As adults, bladder and bowel incontinence is treated as something shameful and unmentionable. We need to deodorize it and hide it away. Yet, when I made jokes in a speech about incontinence products, a woman came to me afterward in tears. It was the first time, she said, that she could see humor in something she'd been made to feel so awful about. That it was so freeing to laugh at herself and her situation, and that I had given her permission to do just that.

I will readily admit I've gone for the laugh, sometimes much to the chagrin of those around me. My kids used to call me 'the sit-down comic' when I was in the wheelchair because of my approach to life.

I see us as having two choices: we hide away what is happening to us or we make light of it. To my way of thinking, hiding things away gives them power. They grow into monsters in the dark. If we laugh at them, they shrink in size. They become just one more flea to flick away. They hold no power, no sway, and no fear. That is the power of humor.

I also tend to make terrible jokes when I am nervous or stressed. I've had more than one nurse or doctor look at me sideways as a result. I just can't help it; it's how I see life and the things happening to me. I shape them into something that amuses me and I share that amusement.

I'll never forget when I went back on my daily injectable drug for MS. The very supportive nurse on the phone asked if I needed someone to come out and re-familiarize me with the injection locations and procedure. I said, "No, thank you, I remember the 'MS Macarena' all too well." Dead silence followed. Then, a very hesitant...

"The *what*???'

I explained to her that I had dubbed the shot locations as my 'MS Macarena'. Imagine the hand motions to that dance. First, two shots in the belly. Then, one in each thigh. Then, one in each upper arm. Then, one on each side of the backside. Hey, MS Macarena!

Made... her... day!

So, I can be angry at my MS. I can be tired of taking a daily injection. Or, I can laugh it off and dance my way through. I'll take humor over grousing any day.

When you care about someone with a chronic illness...

When I was walking one evening with my amazing friends, I heard something I'd never heard before. My friend, Robin, told me she had researched MS when she learned of my relapse. It took a moment for my brain to process that remarkable comment and several other friends added that they had conducted their own bit of research for the same reason. Just because I relapsed, they had taken the time to try and understand MS, without asking me a lot of questions. Now, I wouldn't have minded the questions. But, this effort, this gesture on my behalf, moved me beyond words.

My father, years ago, had done his share of research on my behalf, but this was different. This small gesture meant so much to me. They cared enough to stop their own lives, to see what I was facing and to better understand how they could support me. Then, they joined my

WalkMS team, Barb's MonSter Slayers, and walked beside me.

It's not the big things that people do that stay with you, although grand gestures are nice. It's these small, seemingly insignificant things that go straight to your heart.

The New Normal: Holding Space

As I mentioned before, if you ask me how I am, I am probably going to either say "I'm fine" or "Well, I have pants on and my shoes match, so I'm good." The truth lies somewhere in between... or somewhere else entirely. I have good days. I have bad days. I have awful days. I rarely, if ever, have great days, physically. And, I am not going to get better any time soon. This is my 'new normal'.

I have to be sure that you understand this. At this time, for most of us with chronic illness, getting better is not in the cards. I welcome your prayers and I have hopes of my own. I know you want me to get better. I want to get better. It's what we all hope and pray for. But, honestly, in most moments, I just want to be where I am and have that be okay with you.

This is our new normal, too, for you and I as friends, family, and colleagues. There are days I won't be able to chat on the phone. There are days I won't be able to go out for coffee. There will be weeks you don't hear from me. There will be days I push myself beyond reason, because I just feel the need to do that.

You need to let me do what I can, when I can, and you need to remind me that we are friends beyond my illness. Don't hover but do ask. Don't assume but do show up. I don't always know what is going to happen, even from moment to moment, and your flexibility and sense of humor are very, very welcome.

There is a change in any relationship, when it includes chronic or life-threatening illness. Roles may change. Expectations change, certainly. One important thing anyone can do is to accept those changes and continue to love, without judgment. Offer us not only a safe place to land, when we feel unwell, but also a safe place from which to fly, on good days.

Please don't try to 'fix' us. Don't give us unsolicited and often unwelcome advice on how we can feel better, do better, look better. Don't compare us to other people you know with a chronic illness. Walk beside us, sometimes holding our hand, always holding our hearts.

You have to let us be reckless. I tend to fight using a cane or a wheelchair long past the point of sane reasoning. I used to fall and crack my head open. I used to find myself helpless on the bathroom floor, all because I fought using the cane or wheelchair. You have to let me fall and sometimes you have to let me pull myself back up. And, please don't scold me as I do these things. I know exactly what I'm doing, crazy as it seems to you, and why I'm doing it. You need to trust that I do.

You also have to let me get angry, without telling me to 'hang in there' or 'don't feel that way'. Expressing anger at my body and my illness (or my doctor, on any given day), is a means of getting those feelings out, so that I can get back to living. Telling me not to be angry or not to be sad is not being there for me. Providing a safe supportive place for me to do just that, and then letting me move on, is. And not just when it's about my illness.

As Heather Plett wrote, in *What It Really Means to Hold Space for Someone*: "We have to be prepared to step to the side so that they can make their own choices, offer them unconditional love and support, give gentle guidance when it's needed, and make them feel safe even when they make mistakes."

Plett's article really shows the how's and why's of holding space for those we love, as well as others. "It is something that ALL of us can do for each other – for our partners, children, friends, neighbours, and even strangers who strike up conversations as we're riding the bus to work." The article includes eight tips and is really worth reading... and printing to post on your refrigerator as a reminder.

Helping is not always helpful. I need to repeat that. Helping is not always helpful. When you walk into your friend's home and start cleaning, before you even get, "Hi, how are you?" out of the way, it only serves to make your friend feel inadequate. Don't bulldoze over my feelings. Don't do for me, when I haven't asked you to do anything at all. I mean, seriously, how would you feel if I came into *your* house and started cleaning?

Yes, ask what your friend needs. Offer to do housework, fold laundry, grocery shop (oh dear god, please offer that one) but listen for the real answer. Is your friend saying 'no' out of pride or because he really just wants you to sit and talk to him like a real person? It may take time to get to the truth of this, but it will be worth it for both of you.

Sometimes, you can learn what we need just by the way we talk about what's overwhelming us. And, sometimes, it helps to ask specific questions... *what can I do for you* or *what do you need* are not always the best routes to an answer. I may not be able to verbalize what I need, in response to that general question.

One area a lot of us grapple with is with our speech. Often, trouble finding the right words accompanies cognitive issues that are so common in chronic illness. For me, when you finish my sentence for me, or suggest a word I'm seeking, my brain goes to what you say and I lose my train of thought.

Sometimes, my hands may shake and it may take a moment or two longer to unlock a door or open a container. Or, I turn the lock the wrong way once or twice to get it open. Jumping in and 'rescuing' us may seem like a good idea in the moment. On the other hand, it can often frustrate us even more than our struggle with that key or that word.

The thing is, we know that it's difficult for you to watch us struggling. When you're feeling impatient, we know that. Your sighs are like screams in our ears and that makes it that much more difficult to accomplish our task. In instances when you just genuinely want to help us and relieve us of the stress in that moment, we can end up feeling belittled and insignificant. All this comes at a cost to our self-esteem, however. We ask that you do not try to take from us things we can still do, albeit with some extra effort and frustration.

If you see me struggling or if you hear me say I'm struggling with something, that would be the cue to make a specific offer of help. I may have told you in the past not to help in such moments, and I would ask you to respect that until I change the 'guidelines'. If I haven't done that, ask me specifically "when this happens, what do you want me to do?" and let me tell you.

It's a tricky road to maneuver and I admit that without hesitation. I am difficult to help. But, don't stop trying.

Sticks and Stones...the power of words

The reality of the childhood rhyme is that words can hurt. Words hold power and, once uttered, cannot be taken back. Apologies may be offered, or not, but the words hang in the air and no amount of wishing them away will work.

It is important to recognize that a person in a vulnerable position, such as the one we are in when someone else has to take care of us, can feel a great deal of anger and frustration, as well as impotence. Given our weakened physical resources, we may lash out with words.

It is also important to recognize that the caregiver, being in a position of more power, can also feel frustrated, angry, put upon, and overwhelmed. Those feelings may well become directed at the one being tended to and the words may spill out from time to time.

At a time when I was extremely ill, having trouble breathing, and fearing a relapse had indeed found its way into my life, I was told I was 'useless, lazy and no good' to my supposed partner. The irony of that statement is that I was still doing housework, creating the items we sold in a handmade business, and writing my second novel. Still, the words had an impact on me. As you can see, I will never forget them.

It may well feel that someone is lazy, when they appear well enough to you to do more than they are doing. The thing is, it's not up to you to judge that, and telling them that they are lazy may well cause them to curl up more, rather than to spur them to more activity.

Abuse can come in many forms and verbal abuse is no less damaging than physical abuse. The words enter our brains and then slip into our souls. Even as we recognize the lie in them, we take them in and they can begin to become part of how we see ourselves.

In a time when we all feel compelled to share every thought in our heads on the internet and when we feel that we have the right to express every single opinion we have, we need to also consider that not all thoughts need to be stated out loud. And, that there are consequences to saying what you think.

For every word you speak, there is someone receiving those words on the other end. Be aware that you can hurt or heal, empower or disable, encourage or deflate, by your choice of words.

Caregivers – the unsung heroes

Caregivers, you are my heroes. I know I am difficult and testy and frustrating. I know I make things harder for you than they have to be. I know that, some days, you'd rather be anywhere than here, taking care of me.

I also know that you can experience so much, because of what I'm going through. You sometimes feel helpless, watching me struggle and suffer, often knowing that there is nothing you can do to relieve it.

I know you sometimes feel hopeless, when thinking about what is yet to come and that there is not yet a cure. That you feel trapped and sometimes want to run away. That you feel overwhelmed and alone and paralyzed by it all. I also know you feel angry, at doctors and the world, and sometimes... with me.

Emotions are normal and natural. They are our response to and our way of processing the world and the experiences life brings us. They can be helpful or they can trap us like quicksand.

Your emotions are no less important than mine, in dealing with life and chronic illness. Whether you are a partner, an adult child, a family friend, or a paid caregiver, you cannot pretend you don't feel all the things this relationship does to you.

You absolutely must give yourself your own set of prescriptions. You require time to yourself, away from me and your caregiving responsibilities. Never mind that you love me and do all the things you do out of love. You need time away from me, to rest and rejuvenate. Whether it's a spa day or a day out with friends to play softball or seeing a movie by yourself, you must do this.

You need to talk to someone who is not me. Not just about how you're feeling, either. You need to talk about other things, specifically not related to my illness. You need time and space to just be you.

Self-care, for you, must also include your own physical well-being. Do go work out. Do go walking. Do go to see your own doctors for your own health. Do eat well. Do nourish your own soul.

Sleep. Nap. Read. Garden. Bowl. Clog dance. Whittle. Yodel. Study Gaelic. Be you. The more you care for yourself, the better you'll be able to care for me. The more you care for yourself, the happier and healthier you will be.

If you are a paid caregiver, allow time between patients to regroup. Be sure your time off is truly time off from caregiving, for anyone but yourself. Yes, you get paid for what you do for me (and I'm sure you do not get paid enough), but you deserve time to care for yourself as well.

If you are a parent and a caregiver, remember you are both. You do your child no favors if you do not expect the same behavior from him or her that you do from your children who are not ill. The tendency to go easy on your child or to spoil your child will not serve either of you well. But, do remember to cherish the time you spend together apart from the doctors' appointments and therapy sessions. Do remember to let your child be a child and be a parent. Play games. Eat candy (if that is allowed). Swim in the pool. Build sandcastles. Watch movies. And do all those things together.

If you are an adult child who is his or her parent's (or other relative's) caregiver, remember that these are the people who taught you to use a spoon, ride a bike, read a book, and drive a car. They brought you into this world, changed your diapers, and dried your tears. Treat them with respect and dignity.

If there are issues between you, do not

use the caregiver relationship as a means to repay hurt for hurt. Remove yourself from the issues as much as you can while you are seeing to the duties of caregiving. Reserve conversation and raising those issues to quiet moments of talking or even for a counselor.

If you are a lover, remember to be a lover. Caregiving is one of the most sacred ways of caring for any loved one and that is no less true for you. Preserve dignity, introduce gentle humor, and let touch speak for you when words cannot convey depth of feeling. Hold hands, brush hair, kiss her forehead, stroke his beard, and nibble an ear now and then. Remember what drew you together in the beginning and remind your lover of that from time to time.

If you are a friend who is also a caregiver, try and keep those coffee conversations and shopping trips going, even as you help me live my life. Don't forget what drew you to me as a friend, and keep that friendship going. Step away, when you need to, because I love you for caring for me and I want you to care for yourself, too. And let me be your friend. Share your life and your concerns, your triumphs and your heartbreaks, just as you would if I were well. That you would do that tells me I am not finished yet and I have worth beyond being your patient.

To all caregivers: Do not let others reduce me to an afterthought and, please, do not commiserate about your burdens in front of me. Demonstrate respect for me by not standing and speaking over my head to others.

Speak for me, when I cannot speak for myself, but let my voice be heard.

Shut up and dance with me

By all means, tell us how you are feeling too. Most days, I would probably rather listen to you talk about all you're doing, how you're feeling, what you're dreaming of, than to spend one moment talking about my illness. It doesn't bother me to hear about the things you're struggling with.

It also doesn't bother me to hear all that is going well in your life. I am your friend and I can celebrate your successes without feeling jealous. I can commiserate with you, without feeling put upon. In fact, sharing with me tells me you still consider me a valued friend. That goes a long way to helping me feel whole and valuable.

By all means, ask me how I'm feeling... and accept my answer. And, watch my eyes. I have a friend who lives with chronic illness. I can usually tell a good day from a bad one by her eyes. The smile that doesn't quite reach her eyes is always a good clue. She's often surprised when I tell her I can tell she's not feeling well on a particular day, by the look in her eyes. It's there, if you pay attention.

And, please, by all means, shut up and listen when we want to talk. Please don't tell me how it will all get better, because it may never get better. Because it may well get worse. Don't tell me how brave I am and how strong I am and, heaven forbid, how great I look. Listen, really listen to me. Encourage the tough talk and the tender feelings. Encourage me to get it out there and provide a safe space where I won't feel judged for not being quite that strong now and then.

Then, by all means, don't forget to dance with me. When I recently completed a 5K MS Walk, my friends did one of two things. They walked with me, slowly, to the end, or they met me at the end, having finished before me. They played the theme from "Rocky". They videotaped my tearful step across the finish line. They cheered and hugged and cried right along with me. They posted pictures of our team and our victorious feat.

At no point that day did a single person encourage me to stop. Sure, they checked on me, to see if I was okay as I walked. Yes, one very sweet friend unobtrusively moved behind me on occasion, in case I faltered. But, no one tried to talk me out of finishing. They danced with me, in spirit, as I did something I had no business being able to do.

Let me do too much and celebrate with me when I do. Shut up and dance with me.

When you don't hear from me

There will be times you don't hear from me. I may be too tired or too overwhelmed or too busy with medical appointments. I may be cocooning or honoring my inner introvert. I may feel unwell and be merely trying to get through the day. I may be sleeping or just relishing the quiet. My silence may represent self-care or depression but, whatever the reason, it's not about you.

When you ask me if I'm angry with you or if you've done something wrong, I then have to add taking care of you to my list. Rather, ask me gently if I'm okay and tell me you're there if I need you.

Little things add up

When you are living with chronic illness, little things add up. We don't start from scratch and 'begin again' from the start of each day. Our pile is already high when we start the day and then little things can get to us much more easily than if we were well.

In a foot race, on an oval track, runners

are staggered along the lanes, to ensure they are each off to the same, equal race. It balances the start, but it's up to the runners what they do once the starting gun fires.

When you start the day with chronic illness, you don't get the same consideration from life. Your playing field is never level. So, when it seems that we are easily disturbed, please remember that we started from a very different place than you did that particular day.

Advocacy and support

Part of living with a chronic illness and feeling more in control on a day-to-day basis is through advocacy. On a personal level, you are your own best advocate. Whether it is being proactive in following your paperwork through the disability system or pressing your physician for answers, you are your best advocate because you know your own situation the best. Even someone who loves you, even someone who lives with you, does not fully understand the day-to-day challenges you face.

Advocacy also means speaking up for access, whether it's to your child's classroom or to a community event that is not easily attended when physically challenged. Something as simple as making sure the aisles between the desks allow for a wheelchair means you will be able to attend your child's back-to-school night. Bringing challenges to the attention of community leaders and school personnel not only helps you participate. It opens the conversation, and the door, for others who may not be able to speak up for themselves.

If you live with physical challenges and/or chronic illness, and you have children, teaching them advocacy shows them they have a voice and teaches them how to use it for change. My children have, at times, told store managers the restroom door was too heavy for someone in a wheelchair, spoken to the state legislators about funding research and accessibility, and created handmade items to sell to support the National MS Society. My son, at age twelve, rode a bike 150 miles in two days, for me and to raise money and awareness. My daughter walked the two-day MS Challenge Walk at age ten for the same reason. Now, as adults, they speak up with confidence, about accessibility and social issues.

Learning to advocate for others, at a young age, teaches children compassion, along with a host of other skills. It also offers them a chance to feel more in control of an uncontrollable situation and helps them feel empowered when they might otherwise feel impotent.

On a larger stage, you can advocate for people with chronic illness with regard to local, state, and federal legislation, as well as funding for research and more. Some organizations make this very easy, by having you sign up to help advocate. You can simply send an email when important legislation is being considered. You can help yourself and others without ever leaving home. Remember that each time we lift our voices together, we can be better heard and we can achieve even more.

But, why should you do all this? You may be wondering why you should use your 'spoons' to help others, when it is so hard to just get through the day. There is one very good reason above all the others: because it empowers YOU. The more you accomplish, the more you contribute, the more you look outside yourself just a little, the more powerful you will feel. The more fulfilled you will feel.

You will also come in contact with others doing the same work and facing similar challenges to your own. You will find that you inspire one another, to continue and to grow. Quickly, you can build a community of change around you. Believe me, this will be something you will cherish.

When you ask for help

It is important to ask for help when you need it. When that involves calling a doctor's office, an agency, a foundation, or a government office, remember that there is another human being on the line (hopefully) and to treat them the way you would like to be treated. Even when they do not treat you the same way.

Remember to express your gratitude when someone is kind, supportive, and helpful. Compliment their tender care of your concerns. We often overlook complimenting good care and great service, because we expect it. You could very well make someone's day by simply being grateful.

Consider the other person, on the other end of your request. He or she may have had a day of having to turn down people's requests for assistance. Imagine how it would feel to want to help but be unable to do so. After a day of having to say no to people, you could be hearing the strain of their day when they speak with you.

Consider, too, that people in support positions may be steeling their hearts against the needs that are presented to them day in and day out, as a way of protecting their own feelings. I honestly don't know how they do this, day in and day out. It's much more difficult to be angry at the individual if you consider these things when speaking with them.

I once spoke to someone at the MS Society, who had to tell me that she could not help me find housing. For me, it had already been 'a day' and I broke down in tears. I could hear her tortured response and stopped to ask her if she was okay. I told her that I appreciated all she did for those of us with MS. I thanked her for the job she does (she's a volunteer, by the way) and that I understood that it must be so difficult when she can't help us with the very things we need.

She was floored. No one, in all the time she'd been doing her job, had asked how she was. There is something very wrong with that.

No one likes to be treated badly by office staff or medical staff when we don't feel well. These are the very people who are supposed to be on our side, who are paid to provide 'care'. Likewise, we need to remember others have feelings too.

Adapting to change, and living versus existing

In his novel, *Honesty*, Seth King writes that 'pockets of happiness can be found within misery'. It is essential to remember this. Whether you are struggling with grief and anger, or you are struggling to get your shoes on the correct feet, sometimes we can get bogged down into only seeing the misery or the 'less than' in our lives. We measure the losses and take stock of the changes. It all becomes a matter of survival, just getting through the day.

The problem with that is that you then are simply existing, just getting by. You need to search for that 'happiness within misery' and get back to really living. Will this new life look just like your old one? Maybe, maybe not. To me, that is less important than whether or not you are living versus simply existing.

When I went into remission the second time, the changes were so significant that I felt I needed to mark the event. Ritual is so healing and it focuses our gratitude so profoundly. In our modern world, we often overlook the value of rites of passage and ceremony. So, I created my own ritual, my own rite of passage, to becoming a walking being once more.

Part of that ceremony included claiming a new name, for my rebirth. Part of that name included the Welsh word 'gorfoleddu', which means 'joy in the midst of or in spite of sorrow'. It reminded me of the bitter-sweet dichotomy that is honored in the first night of Passover, that we must always recognize both the bitter and the sweet of life. And, it reminds me to dance in spite and in the midst of sorrow.

Life, written in pencil

Day planners are a must, when you have a chronic illness (more on this in Tangible Advice). But, equally important, are pencils. Because life as you know it will now be written in pencil. Erasable pencil. Changeable pencil.

Other than those pesky, yet oh-so-important doctors' appointment, you will now have to consider writing any plans you make in pencil. There will be days you just can't do what you planned to do. This is so hard to accept, particularly in the beginning when you are still reeling from your diagnosis and all that internet research you've done.

Learn to say 'no'

While I will never, ever advise you to use your chronic illness as an excuse for anything, I will say, and probably repeat more than once, that it has some added gifts. One of them is learning boundaries. I never cease to be amazed at the number of us who 1) have been diagnosed with a chronic illness and who also 2) have no personal boundaries. Someone should probably do a study on this but, for now, learn to recognize that you may possess this combination of traits. If so, it's time to learn to say 'no'.

I'm sure we all do this to some extent, but, for me, I was a card-carrying, tee-shirt-wearing member of the codependent council of the worst sort. I had no idea how to say no to things I really didn't want to do. I would be wracked with guilt at the mere thought. I'm still working to overcome this tendency.

In business, it's important to do those things that move your business forward. Things that have a reasonable return on investment, whatever that might be. It is essential that you know how to judge these things, before making decisions and investing your time and talent.

The same is no less true of our health and well-being. Truthfully, whether or not you have a chronic illness, you should set strong, reasonable boundaries around things like family time, personal time, and creative time. We, especially women, have been taught that to say no to someone is to be selfish.

Well, I'm here to tell you that it's ok to say no, selfish or not. If you can't do something, you can't do it. If you don't want to waste a spoon on it, don't waste a spoon on it. Do those things that move you forward, either in terms of health or happiness. Invest in the people you love and who love you. That's where your return on investment will come from.

So, you might be asking, how do you learn to say no? I'll give you one example:

I had a neighbor who began a daily ritual of calling me, before she left to start her day. The call consisted of dumping every ounce of drama in her life onto me, and there was a lot of it. She would, for lack of a better visual, offer up her daily 'verbal vomit' each and every day and then go off to do her own thing. That left her feeling relieved and me feeling, well, dumped on.

At first, because I was so incredibly codependent, I had no idea what was happening and what it was going to me. I would realize how stressed I was as I began my own day, but I didn't put the two things together. One day, like the proverbial lightning bolt, it hit me. She was using me to relieve her own pressures, and I was standing there with hands wide open to take it all on.

The next day, I summoned the gumption to tell her I couldn't talk any longer, as soon as she began to dump. She spluttered a bit and tried again. I fought the urge to waver and said that I was truly sorry but that I had to get off the phone. She tried each morning for the rest of that week to dump on me. Each day, I stood fast and politely said I wasn't able to talk. She finally gave up.

Setting boundaries is a difficult thing to do, as is saying no, when we haven't been taught how to do it. I recommend finding one thing that gives your stomach the willies and begin there. Find the kindest, gentlest, politest way to extricate yourself from the 'thing'. Hold fast, as resistance to your 'no' becomes apparent. Step up your own stance as needed to see it through until the no is accepted.

Each time you to do this, it really does get a little easier. Practice may not make perfect; it does make you better at things. You may never be a pro at it; I'm certainly not. But, you can improve, and that's all you really need to do.

Learn to say 'maybe'

Remember that pencil? This is where that comes in handy. Welcome an invitation to something you really want to do and let them know, in no uncertain terms, that you will *try* to be there. Work the 'maybe' for those things you really want to do, but don't necessarily have to do, and learn the difference. People will learn to accept this as you go, if they care about you and really want you to participate. They will also learn a valuable lesson in chronic illness.

Consider putting items in your planner with a color-coding system. For example, items that are 'have to do' can be one color (even a dot of color beside the entry), 'want to do' can be a second color, and 'might do' can be a third color. This is a good reminder for you when you start to feel obligated but really aren't. And, having to choose the color helps you think about how important some of these obligations are. It's another practice that can become second nature and 'rewire' the way you think about things.

An aside about 'the maybe': it can become far too easy to give in and stay in. Be sure that your maybe doesn't become a no because it's easier not to go out. That can become a habit that is difficult to break later on. Remember to live your life, while you're living with illness.

Learn to say 'yes'! New ways to do old things

One of the things that has always brought me joy is gardening. I have never lost the wonder of that five-year-old girl watching seeds grow into seedlings, and I am still in awe of how a huge, fragrant tomato plant laden with ripe tomatoes grew from one tiny seed. It is a tie to my parents, who grew vegetables and zinnias, and to my children, who loved having gardens of their own as they grew up.

Gardening is good for the soul, in connecting us back to the earth, the sun, the rain, and the animals with whom we share this world. It is good for the body, in both providing nourishing food, and exercise and fresh air. It can also be challenging when one walks with crutches or moves about in a wheelchair.

Because gardening is so much a part of who I am, I found ways to keep doing it. I found an accessible greenhouse (sadly no longer available) and cut down the legs of my potting bench so I could reach it from a seated position. I used telescoping trowels, claws, and grabbers to plant, pick, and weed. Lightweight hoses allowed me to water, and planting in pots allowed me access to all of my plants.

On days I can't garden, I can sip a cup of herbal tea and peruse gardening catalogs. I can discuss gardening in online groups. I can pin items online that I dream about doing in a garden. I can buy a rooted basil plant at the supermarket and cook with fresh-picked basil. I can stroll through the farmer's market to experience the scents, textures, and tastes that I love. There are ways to connect to things we love, even when we aren't physically up to doing them.

As I've mentioned before, artists who live with physical challenges use their mouths to hold paintbrushes and colored pencils. Adaptive equipment in vehicles keeps us driving, just like crutches keep us moving. Whatever your passion, before the chronic illness, it is still your passion. Whatever your gift, your talent, you can still pursue it.

So, now, if your passion was basketball or ballet, you're thinking I have no idea what I'm talking about. But, you see, I do. If you cannot play basketball (although there are wheelchair leagues), you can coach. You can encourage others faced with challenges to stay active or you can coach children to play. I taught both my children to catch, throw, and hit a baseball, all while I was in the wheelchair, and took them to Phillies games.

Dance is your passion? Teach. Mentor. Dance in your wheelchair, because I would love to see someone stage a wheelchair ballet. Do old things in new ways. Adapt your passion to your life and continue to do all the things you love in some way, to nourish your soul.

Learn to say 'yes': new things

As I wrote earlier, this is a great time to try new things. We need to sometimes search for joy and there is no better time than when we are living with chronic illness. There are things lurking in the dusty corners of your soul that you've always longed to do. Break 'em out, dust 'em off, and give 'em a try.

Trace that family ancestry you always wanted to know about and learn upon whose shoulders you stand. Write that novel that has been burning to be written or begin research on that non-fiction work that the world is waiting for. Paint that sunset or that abstract, or try your hand at pastels or watercolors or charcoal. Bake all those things you never attempted before. Learn auto repair. Take up bocce. Start a walking club or chess club.

Want to travel but feel it would be too much for you? Research places to go and start a dream book of brochures, maps, history and more. Watch videos about those places and movies set there. Read books by authors born there and poems written by native poets. Immerse yourself and travel that way.

Always wanted to learn more or get a degree? Do it! Online courses are readily available and offer a chance to learn things just because we want to. You often do better in formal education later in life because you bring so much more to the classes. There are so many new things to do and learn, this is no time to stop doing just that and the perfect time to start.

Make the most of the good days, self-care on the bad days

I often point out that, when you live with chronic illness, you take assessment each morning when you wake up, to see what works and what isn't working quite so well. Then, you go about your day, making adjustments. You make the most of the good days, often overdoing it, much to the chagrin and concern of those who love you. You try to squeeze it all in on those days, to get it all done.

It is so important to know, when you're having a bad day, that you're allowed to have a bad day. You must give yourself permission to take care of yourself. Your body is telling you what it needs and you need to listen to it.

These are the rough days mentally for me, the days when I feel as if I'm giving in to the MS. I feel awful cancelling lunch dates with friends. I'm disappointed that I can't attend my events. I hate relying on my daughter to bring me meals or help me to the bathroom. And, the entire time, friends and family are telling me that it's okay. That I'm allowed to take it easy when I need to. And, that they are here for me. My daughter always points out that I would do all of it for her in a heartbeat, yet I have so much trouble accepting the help for myself.

Self-care is important, vital, and it needs to be one of the tools you employ. Mothers feel guilt for taking time for themselves. Fathers feel they are not the strong, reliable men they were taught to be. As a parent, you are also teaching a life lesson. Our children emulate us, far more than they listen to us. If we demonstrate that it is never acceptable to take time for ourselves, they will learn that lesson. I see this in my own adult children.

Adult children feel they are letting down their parents, if they cannot be the caregiver for the day. But, the truth is, you need the day or days to take care of yourself. You are no less important than anyone else. And, as someone vital to your family or to your workplace, you need to do what you have to for yourself.

This is yet another prescription you can fill for yourself. Permission granted.

The internet as a lifeline

I am old enough to remember life before the internet and to be fully aware of its impact on our daily lives. Like all things, it has its benefits and its drawbacks. Let's face it, when you research symptoms online, you can scare the pants off yourself. You can also get caught up in scams or stalked or any number of things from which you would protect yourself.

Yet, one of those vital lifelines can come from being connected to the 'net. I have made friendships that I value so highly and reconnected with family members after many years. I mention my friend Lynne in the 'gifts' chapter for this very reason. She became a lifeline for me and is a friend of the heart. We even had a chance to meet in person, as I have with several other internet friends, and that has only deepened our connection.

The internet offers places to join groups that can offer support and information. Facebook alone has thousands of groups founded by people with similar interests, experiences, and, yes, illnesses. Charity and support organizations offer websites with information and connection. The internet is a place to learn, to share, and to connect.

While online connections should not replace in-person human ones, they can be there for you when you cannot physically be out and about. You should protect yourself no less vigorously online than you do in 'real life', especially because it is so easy for someone to misrepresent who they really are when online. And, you should never follow the 'if it's on the internet, it must be true' line of reasoning.

The internet also offers a great means to stay in touch with others when you can't or don't want to see them. Email, private messaging, online posting… these all offer a way to let others know where you are, how you are, and to stay in touch, when you feel it's too much to go out or invite people into your home. Again, it shouldn't replace real live connection when you can do that. But, it keeps you from feeling isolated when you can't.

"Morning song"

Music speaks to our souls on a level that goes beyond words. Yes, the lyrics stay with us. I can remember lyrics to songs from three decades ago, better than I can remember what I had for dinner last week. But, the music itself, that is the song of the spheres, the Oran Mor. It is our heartbeat, reflected back to us. Slow and pulsing or fast and furious, music can reflect what we're feeling or it can inspire us to new heights.

It's that second part I'm going for here. Like most people, I have a morning routine. Most of it is what you'd expect. Some days, even that is not possible, due to fatigue or other MS symptoms. Yet, there is one part of the routine I never miss. That is my morning song.

For me, it is Rachel Platten's *Fight Song*, along with Cher's *You Haven't Seen the Last of Me'*. These two songs never fail to pump me up, get my soul dancing, and even me actually dancing on better days. I may be dancing in my chair, but I am dancing nonetheless.

I sing them for me. I sing them for the world to know I'm neither down nor out. I sing them for those who didn't believe in me. I sing them for those who do believe in me. And, I sing them to make them come true, on those days when they might not be.

Each of us usually has a song that never fails to lift our spirits or to make our souls dance. If you don't have one, I really suggest you find one. And, it may change from time to time, just as we change.

Every single morning, especially if you have a few moments all by yourself, put that morning song on and listen, sing, and dance in any way you can. And, I mean, really sing it. OWN it. If you have to, play it while you drive to work or your doctor's appointment. But, do it. Take it in, let it fill you, music and lyrics, and belt out that baby. Croon like no one is listening (it really helps if they're not), and give it all you've got. Imagine you're on stage and the stadium or auditorium echoes back your passion, your tears, even the break in your voice. Sing to the Universe and to the angels. Give it your all.

Even if you don't have a chronic illness or even if it's a 'good day', make this part of your routine. I talk about this all the time with the aspiring authors with whom I work, because repeated good habits help offset any ingrained bad habits. Get your morning song playing right before you get started each day, and you start on a high note!

Have a dream you are trying to make come true? Morning song before you start. Bad day, physically or emotionally? Morning song as soon as you get up. Heck, before you get up. Dreaded meeting at work? Morning song before going in. Facing hours and hours in an MRI tube? Morning song before (and if possible, during).

Get yourself a morning song, sing it like nobody's business as you start your day, and carry yourself through the day on it. Ride that particular wave to a better day.

Tools of the trade

If your physical abilities change, you may need some adaptive tools to assist you in continuing to live your life well. I, in the interest of full disclosure, do not accept this well. I fight against using canes, walkers, and wheelchairs, in particular, far beyond anything close to reason.

Having said that, I do eventually relent, in order to keep going and going safely. So, I have a few suggestions for you.

When selecting a cane, particularly in the beginning, consider a collapsible one. This allows you to have the cane with you at all times, in a handy dandy pouch, so it's there when you need it and tucked away when you don't. These are often lightweight, so less taxing to use, and adjustable for your height. They also come in a variety of lovely designs and colors.

No, I'm not crazy. Consider your cane a

fashion accessory, and you'll be more likely to use it. Why settle for boring black (though it goes with everything) when you can have purple butterflies, blue tropical flowers, or woodgrain? Some even have flashlights, for the guy who has to have every single nifty gadget in his life. Or a vintage 'walk stick' might be just the thing to help you feel more dapper.

And, see that lovely handle? Turn the cane over and use it as a hook, so you don't have to bend over and risk falling, especially in the bathroom or kitchen. Lift charger cords to you, rather than bending to them, and retrieve that pair of pants that dropped to your ankles. Make the most of every part of each tool you use.

Grabbers are a huge help for anyone who struggles physically. And, for short people like me, they are a lifesaver. Again, you can use the grabber to pick things up, so you don't bend over and risk greater injury. You can reach things without climbing on stools or counters or couches. And, you can get to inaccessible areas.

An added bonus is that you can do other cool things with grabbers. My favorite is to garden with them. I can take a plant out of the pot, grab the dirt ball gently with the grabber, and settle the plant into the waiting hole in the soil (which I dug with a telescoping trowel), all from my wheelchair.

Telescoping garden tools are out there,

and they keep you gardening and growing and enjoying all that comes with that particular hobby. If there are not adapted tools for your favorite past time, make your own. Don't give up and never give in.

If you use a walker or a wheelchair, add a bag to help you carry things around with you. My children always called the pocket on the back of my wheelchair my 'magic pocket'. I had so many things in there, that moms often have handy, and took those everywhere with me. And I had my grabber hanging on the back too, so I could reach anything I needed.

Shower chairs are a huge help, if you can't stand too long or if there is a chance you might get lightheaded in the shower. Keep all your toiletries in a shower caddy right by your side. And, consider transferring shampoo, condition, and body wash to smaller, easier-to-handle containers.

Car handles are something I wished I'd invented. These handles slip into the loop on your car's door frame and give you a great support when standing up out of your car. Then, you just pull it back out to close the car door.

Slide or transfer boards are another great tool. These are highly polished, smooth boards that allow you to slide from one seat to another. Whenever we went to an amusement park, the transfer board came along for the ride. I could slide onto the seats on the rides from my wheelchair, and back again when the ride was over. Wheelchair to car, wheelchair to shower chair, wherever I need to transfer, the board allowed for easy movement and far less risk of falling and injury.

Covering the cost

One of the issues with adaptive tools may be the cost. They are often too expensive for us, no matter how much we may need them. If your insurance doesn't cover them, and it often doesn't, look into other funding sources.

If you have a diagnosis, find an organization, foundation, or 'society' that helps and supports those living with a particular illness. If you are undiagnosed or your particular situation has not specific group, local Lions Clubs or other groups may be able to help. This is one of those areas where asking for help can have a huge impact on your daily life.

Another thought

As much as you may fight against these adaptive tools, if you're anything like me, or if you accept them more gracefully, don't forget others may be affected by them as well. If you have children in your life, let them try out your tools and test drive your wheelchair. I had no idea, until recently, that my daughter felt fear when she first saw my cane, walker, and wheelchair all those years ago. I've learned from her that allowing her to touch and play with these tools gave her a chance to overcome that fear.

It may help if they can decorate your tools with stickers or even name them. If the purple wheelchair had arrived that one day, it would have been 'the purple people eater'. When the red one showed up instead, my kids pointed out that it matched my hair, so it became 'the Mom Mobile'.

Ask them to think of ways you can use the tools. Teach them that it's not okay to take another's adaptive tools without asking, but that it is ok to ask questions about them and to still help us when we need it. Help them adjust, as you yourself are adjusting.

To tell or not to tell...

...that's a big question. You know how you felt when you were told you have Multiple Sclerosis or Rheumatoid Arthritis or Lupus or whatever diagnosis you've received. It may have been a shock, because of a sudden onset of the condition or because you'd never consider the possibility. It may have been a relief, after years of trying to figure out what was going on.

Yet, when the dust settled, you were the same person you'd been before those words were uttered. No different, just a name for the weirdness going on in your body. But, now, with whom do you share this information?

Seems simple, yes? Surely you tell your spouse or significant other. Hold that thought. Surely you tell your parents and your children, siblings, friends. After all, they all have your best interests at heart. And, of course, they will now understand that what you've been experiencing is real, has a name, and that doctors believe you. And, then, there's your employer.

I say 'hold that thought' because nothing about chronic illness is simple. If I were in a loving, truly committed relationship, my partner would have been sitting next to me, holding my hand while I heard the diagnosis. He would have already known I was struggling with symptoms, been scared *for* me, and shared my tears and fears as I began to research what I was facing, what *we* were facing together.

I wasn't in a loving, committed relationship when this recent relapse hit. I was with someone who stated that he probably wouldn't stay with me if I did relapse. So, telling him would end the relationship. For me, that's not a relationship I want to be in and I had enough to deal with, without having to negotiate the truth. Because not telling him would be like lying, right?

The ideal family would also be loving, supportive, and understanding. Not all families are like that, though. Choices of what to share, how much, and when are something we all have to think about.

Employers? This can be a minefield. You may feel that loyalty to your employer compels you to be honest with, say, your immediate supervisor. Not telling him or her feels like a lie. And, what if they find out later, that you didn't tell them? Again, it's that pesky sin of omission.

Yet, watch their eyes when you do. Yes, you are the same employee you were five minutes ago. Unfortunately, they may now see you as a liability, be calculating what this will cost the department and the company, and be thinking back to all the times your illness may have already affected your work. Or, they may offer their hand, to hold yours, and ask how you are feeling, if you're in any pain, and if there is anything they can do. How to know for sure is the minefield I referenced earlier.

Please don't misunderstand; I'm not saying all partners, families, and employers are going to be unsupportive. What I am saying is think before you share, understand why you feel the need to share with this particular person, at this particular time. Look back over the relationship that you've had, to key moments where you might have needed support.

- How did that go?
- Did you receive what you needed?
- Did it come up later, during times of stress or conflict?
- Why do you feel the need to tell them right now?

Start where you know love and trust are strong. Start slowly, revealing what you now know. Lay the groundwork for an ongoing support system of love and caring.

The gift of chronic illness

Yes, you read that correctly. It is a gift. You may not think so and you may be thinking I'm crazy. Just hear me out.

In our society, we are taught to face challenges as they come our way and, once defeated, we look back to see the lesson, the silver lining. You can't do that while fighting the good fight, right? So very wrong. What a waste of precious time and what a waste of what is right in front of us!

I knew, even as I struggled through my second relapse, that one of the most precious gifts of my MS was more time with my parents, particularly with my dad. Time I would not have had, if I were well. Time my children would not have experienced, if I were well. That meant, I knew in those moments that they were gifts. How sad would it have been for me, if I'd only realized that after I lost them both in the same summer?

Through the fledgling internet, I made friends. One friend appeared when my sister's friend asked her church to pray for me. Lynne not only prayed; she reached out to me. We have since met in person and correspond to this day. Others, I met through Myspace and Facebook; some of them I have also met in person, others connect through posts and PMs. They are many and they are always close at hand when I need them. I have learned from them and leaned on them, and celebrated life's joys with them.

Another gift of my illness was and is the honing of my passion for writing. Once a method used to cope with unbearable pain, it has evolved into so much more. Had I not written then, because of my symptoms, you would not be reading this book now. I would not know so many of the people that I do and some of them may not have been inspired to publish their own writing.

My children would tell you that it was a gift for them as well. Yes, I missed ball games because I couldn't be out in the heat. I missed art shows, because the gallery wasn't accessible. But, they learned that you can still do what you love, even with a chronic illness. That you can fight for what you believe in and make a difference. That you grow, as you fight, and that you can face anything with the right people beside you.

They learned how to love someone no

matter what happens to them, through thick and thin. They learned to speak up when injustice looms and they learned to do all they can to change things when they are wrong. They found out they were made of fire and steel and unbreakable spirit. And that anything is possible.

After the Miracle

"Impossible situations can become possible miracles."
~ Robert H. Schuller ~

Pretty much everyone accepts that major upheavals in our lives, such a job loss, death, childbirth, etc., affect those around us while they also affect us. Major changes often shift paradigms and roles. Few have been exempt from such changes in their lives and most people can relate to them on some level.

What few people seem to understand, however, is that a miracle in one's life is just as unwieldy a change as any other. I have seen that many marriages do not survive the ravages of chronic diseases such as Multiple Sclerosis. Mine did not survive the absence of my illness.

A drastic change such as the one I underwent - a complete shifting of my consciousness, spirituality, my very essence - is a miraculous event. I walk with new legs, see with new eyes, feel with new skin, and have a sense of joy and wonder about everything in the world I inhabit. My hands are constantly busy creating new things and trying new hobbies. Those who shared my world and supported me through my illness could now share in the miracle of my remission. I offered that chance with open arms. Not all in my life, however, wished to share that joy.

Roles were changed. Independence replaced need. Excuses for failure vanished with my pain. Pretext for another suddenly sat unused alongside my old wheelchair. The world became my shiny new pearl, and it may have been new and beautiful in my eyes, but those very awe-filled moments became a source of anger and resentment for someone else. Removing the pearl from the oyster kills the creature that formed it. So, too, my old life died with my new.

There is counseling for job loss. There are new parent support groups and grief support groups. There is no support group for those whose lives have been changed by joy, blessing, and wonder. There is no change without cost. There is no healing, it seems, without some pain somewhere. Who'd have thought such a miracle would be tempered by sorrow or even fear?

Be aware that, as you achieve even the smallest amount of success with regard to remission of your chronic illness or curing of your disease, there may be those who are skeptical or who attempt to hold you back. In fairness, they are probably concerned for you and are only acting out of love for you. They may fear you are only in remission and do not want you to get your hopes up too high. Or, they may be acting out of their own need to keep the status quo and their own place secure.

Whichever is the case, it is important to acknowledge that changes in your own life, whether positive or negative, affect those around you. Offer to listen. Hear them out. Acknowledge their fears and concerns. But, do not forget that anyone who loves you truly would want you to be happy.

There is life after diagnosis of chronic illness. So, too, there is life after remission or the miracle of healing. After 45 years in New Jersey, I moved to California. Instead of the Jersey Shore and the Pine Barrens in my backyard, I have the Pacific and Los Angeles. I have found peace and safety and new beginnings in California, and my now-grown children and I look forward to all the future holds. I have earned my first college degree, published more than nine books and am working as an editor, formatter, and public speaker, as well as starting my own publishing company and magazine.

I am living proof that change is not only possible but necessary. I am also living proof that we can survive anything, change anything, become anything... if we only believe. The only limitations in life are the ones we impose upon ourselves.

Yes, life will often show up with new challenges that we never saw coming. Yes, our bodies may limit us in some ways. They may force us to change the way we do things, but we can still do them. We need only take the time to dream of what we want, imagine what might be, see it all as possible, and then create the circumstances that bring those dreams to life. Dreams are as adaptable as we are.

"Survivor" to "Phoenix"

Remember when I wrote earlier about getting stuck? One place I've seen people get stuck is the 'survivor' stage. I don't mean just surviving, versus living. I'm referring to that point where you've overcome and have 'survived' the storm.

Whether it's surviving a life-threatening illness or surviving a domestic violence (or other life-altering) situation, we feel a great sense of relief when the sun finally begins to shine again. Yet, we can get stuck in that place, that survivor mode, just as we can get stuck in the stages of grief.

I'm not suggesting that you don't celebrate the positive changes in your life. You've earned them, and we should always celebrate the good things we experience. I am suggesting, however, that there is a stage beyond that of survivor.

This is the phoenix stage. The butterfly stage, perhaps, if you prefer that metaphor. Imagine the butterfly staying in the cocoon, because she's accomplished that amazing change from caterpillar to 'survivor'. She could stop there, but why should she?

Instead, you can break free of the cocoon and move on to become all you can be. You can emerge, spread your new wings, and fly to new heights. Whatever it is that you survive, whatever it is that you overcome, the world needs you to share that strength and power and positive message.

Just as I written about not 'suffering' from your illness but actually living within in, I'm suggesting that you continue on from being a survivor, after the miracle. Burst into flame, emerge from the ashes, and fly free.

*Get off processed foods, salt, and sugar.
Eat fresh, nutritious food, prepared as closely to its original form as possible. Remove toxins from your home and environment as much as possible. Drink filtered water but stay away from artificial sweeteners and colors.

*Get a day planner and use it for everything. Include phone numbers with appointments, so you don't have to look them up. Put patient ID numbers or other important information in them, so it's at your fingertips all the time (just don't lose it). Make notes of important phone calls so you know who you spoke with when. Color code appointments for 'have to' versus 'want to' versus 'maybe can'. Keep the old ones as an easy way to look up past appointment dates, etc.

*To-do lists: help with memory and feeling a sense of accomplishments. Remember, write in pencil. And check off all you've accomplished, no matter how mundane. Some days, doing the laundry or taking a shower is worth a gold medal.

*Take someone you trust implicitly with you to doctor's appointments... Good news? They can celebrate with you. Not so good news? They can hold your hand. Bad news? They can drive home. They can take notes, so you can just listen. They can ask the questions your mind is too scattered to ask. They can grab the appointment card and remind you to put it in your planner They can confirm for you that the doctor wasn't listening to you or isn't a good fit for you. Grab a cup of coffee afterward and rehash the appointment, to make sure you got everything straight.

*Assess each morning and evening what's working that day and what is not. Adjust your plans accordingly. Congratulate yourself on what you accomplished. Laundry? Grocery shopped? Wrote the next great novel? A lot of small things adds up just as quickly as one big thing. Give yourself credit where credit is due.

*Begin and end with gratitude. The rougher the day, the more important this exercise is. Find at least three things each night to be grateful for. They are there; you just have to look for them.

*Be your own best advocate and authority on your illness/wellness. Never stop researching, learning, verifying, and asking more questions. Try things that make sense to you; skip things that don't.

*Work for change, do something to move a cure forward, advocate for yourself and for others.

*Participate in awareness and fundraising walks (or other events for your diagnosed illness). Fundraise and be there, even if it's to cheer on others at the finish line.

*Focus on what you can do. It keeps your outlook more positive.

*Forgive yourself for what you can't do. It's okay. Let go and move on.

*Find new things to try. Learning and growing are an essential part of a happy, fulfilled life. Every day that you learn something new is a good day.

*Pull out old passions. You have gifts and talents that make life worth living and help you feel accomplished.

***Do not ever stop dreaming and planning.** This helps keep helplessness and hopelessness at bay.

***Journaling helps you identify your emotional and physical state.** It shows changes that could signal improvement or a need for intervention. And, it gives you an outlet when you may not have one. Highlight accomplishments in one color and dreams/goals in another color. When you feel the need to focus on one or the other, it makes them easier to locate in your journal.

***Get a morning song** (or two) and make it part of your routine. And then dance like it's nobody's business but your own.

December 25, 2011...

Tonight, I've had the strangest experience, and that is saying something given all the experiences I've had over my lifetime. Many of my friends here will be aware that I have been through a transformation that continues to this moment. I've always seen transformation as something that moves you forward, that evolves you to a new and different place than you've ever been.

So, what do you call it when you call it when you go back? *When you are suddenly and instantly and irrevocably swept backward through time (a lot of time) to a place before? What do I do now that I'm here?*

This moment came as the result of a day of downloading all of my personal CDs onto a new .mp3 player. It really was a journey down memory lane for me today, for I rarely get to listen to my own music, and it is one of the precious things I relinquished over the years in the name of peace and harmony among residents in my home.

Each CD holds precious memories. Each one transferred is like reclaiming a very important part of just who I am.

But, when the shelf was empty of CDs, on thing remained... an old worn-out broken cassette tape. I don't even remember bringing it to CA with me, though I obviously did. I haven't had a way to play it in a very, very long time, so why would I have brought it? I looked it up on YouTube and hit 'play'. What happened next may be beyond my ability to describe...

It was like in the movies when someone is swept back in time, only it was a sweeping backward of my soul rather than my physical self. Everything from the last three decades was ripped away, leaving only that girl who once was. My heart feels such pain and joy all at the same time, as if it has ripped open and all the festering jagged thorns of abuse and chaos were pulled out all at once. The pain of this experience is really beyond my description because it goes beyond the physical. I cannot stop what is happening to me. The feeling of being back inside myself 'before' is beyond words. And, yet, I am writing to try and *understand it.*

It is certainly not a coincidence that music is responsible for this experience. I know music is an expression of something much deeper, something that tunes our souls to the cosmos, something that joins and binds us. Music is the great Oran Mor to which and through which we are all connected. I know that this particular music comes from that time before, and so it had the power to transport me back. I cannot help but think of the name I took five years ago and it's meaning of "joy in the midst of or as a result of sorrow". Life is like that, after all, if we look carefully enough.

So, I guess I'll go reintroduce myself and get reacquainted...

I woke up one June morning in 2016, completely free of MS. Sadly, this wasn't like the end of my second relapse. I was not free of chronic illness nor any of my symptoms. The day before, my newest neurologist informed me that I don't have MS and that I never did. That I'd been once again misdiagnosed... this time, for eighteen years. That every single doctor, specialist, and radiologist had it wrong all along. It's difficult to describe my emotions at this point.

On one hand, I am thrilled. No one wants to have Multiple Sclerosis. I'd been fighting the monster for decades. It was news anyone would be happy to hear.

On the other hand, I was the same person struggling with the same symptoms that I was before he'd walked into the room. Now, however, those symptoms were once again nameless, faceless. I was back to fighting in the dark, after two decades of thinking I knew my opponent. I'd been fighting a doppelganger, a shadow, a ruse. Someone was wrong eighteen years ago and everyone else had towed the line since.

That second hand? That meant I would begin it all again... the testing, poking, prodding, shocking, scanning. That, for the third time in thirty years, I had no idea what was causing my symptoms and every medical test known to man was going to begin again.

It meant that I would no longer be under the umbrella of the MS Society, for support and for advocacy. I would not be able to call on them in times of need, nor would I be able to represent them as a speaker or advocate with MS. I could not apply for disability (no diagnosis, no prognosis), housing assistance, or any other program.

So, here I am again, swept back to the beginning, to an earlier set of circumstances. This cannot be a coincidence, either. And, now, rereading the above piece I wrote five years ago, I think that is exactly where I am supposed to be. Swept back to the beginning, to who I was before. Before illness, and diagnosis before abuse, before divorce, before compromising who I am over and over and over again. It is time to begin again in so many ways.

It is hard to believe that I am back where I started from, for the third time. I'm back to 'chasing my tail' for a diagnosis and feeling at this point as if one may never appear. It's like boxing with a ghost; you can never land a punch. I'm back on my surfboard, riding waves of grief and anger, even as I work to find my footing and make lemonade from this latest batch of lemons.

Because I do just that, even as I'm angry and uncertain, I am no less determined to win this fight. I've decided that I shall name this unnamed neurological illness 'Fred'. Why? Because Fred is a ninety-pound weakling, a bully, and a liar. He's a cheater and a low-life. Sometimes, he holds on tight and wears me down. Other times, I can beat Fred to a pulp.

Fred has many faces, even some masks, but everyone who has an undiagnosed, life-altering chronic illness knows him. Like all bullies, Fred is a coward who hides in the shadows. By using his name, we can call him out into the light and bop him right in the nose, until he goes down for the count.

As my friend Robin Nieto says, having a diagnosis gives you permission to feel what you feel. People hear the diagnosis and say, 'ok, yes,

I see. You *are* actually ill'. When your symptoms have no name, it's as if they are not legitimate.

She has been struggling with the same issue I am now, as of the writing of this book, but I assure you that she struggles no less with a nameless monster than she would if she had a diagnosis. (see her upcoming book "How I Fought... Like a Girl").

Robin and I are part of the silent undiagnosed. There are no foundations or societies for us. There are no walks or dance marathons to raise funds for our support. There are no ribbons or awareness PSAs. There are few advocacy groups.

We are invisible. We are on the fringes. We are struggling to be seen and heard and diagnosed, and to defeat Fred once and for all.

In that light, I propose a ribbon campaign to bring us together. A sheer ribbon, because there is no name or color for what we have and because we feel so invisible. I propose we take that rug being pulled out from under us and turn it into a flying carpet.

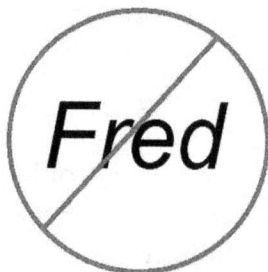

This Glorious Life

During the writing of this book, the rug was pulled out from under me when my diagnosis went from 'MS' to 'you have a neurological disease but we really don't know what it is'. I sat stunned, reeling, and wishing for my dad's hand to hold. He'd been there for all the moments that led up to my MS diagnosis and was there for me afterward.

It was no coincidence that my sister felt the draw to pull out a piece my father had written following his own diagnosis with Myasthenia Gravis. She had her own reasons for needing my dad's guidance that day. That she told me she did also meant that I, too, could have that again.

It was the first time since he wrote it that I read this particular work. I don't remember my dad as someone who processed his life through writing, the way I do, but he clearly felt the need to this one time. I feel the need to put all this in perspective for you, before you read it, so you can truly understand the power in this essay for me.

My parents were both born in 1928, were both 'Depression Babies'. My father grew up within a home that saw a loving family who shared its home with alcoholism. Some shared that tendency with their father; others, like my dad, were determined to make a very different life for their own families.

My mother had a very different experience but was equally affected by the world around her and the worldview of her family. Together, these two people created a family very different than the ones in which they'd been raised.

I will wax poetic about them here, but I assure you that I know my parents were flawed and human. It's not perfection that set them apart, far from it. It's what they accomplished within those flaws that I admire so much and so wish to emulate.

My parents were what my father always described as 'quiet Christians'. He didn't proselytize and only preached when invited to do so as a lay speaker. They both taught Sunday School, her to preschoolers, him to adults. He not only sang in the church choir; he also went to nursing homes to offer hymn sings and comfort to the residents.

They both served their community, in different ways, and those ways inspire me even today. When my dad lost his job due to a quota, he talked to us about living your beliefs and that, if one claims to believe in something, one must be willing to sacrifice in support of those beliefs. When a well-known host of a popular local children's show moved into our neighborhood and tried to convince neighbors not to sell to people of color, in the 1960's, my parents stood firm against her and we welcomed an integrated neighborhood surrounding our home.

My parents were good neighbors and were friends of the first order. Members of their wedding party attended their funerals, having been friends for more than sixty years. They were devoted parents. They were devoted daughter and son to both of their parents. And, they were devoted to one another.

When I first sought a diagnosis for my emerging symptoms in 1983, I saw my mother's rheumatologist. At the time, he said that it wasn't *if* I had some sort of autoimmune or systemic illness; it was more a matter of what it was and when it would hit full force. Why? Because:

- My mother had been diagnosed with Sclerodermatomyositis, an uncommon overlap syndrome which caused her horrific

pain, swelling in her joints, and more.
- My mother's mother had Lupus
- My mother's father had Arterial Lateral Sclerosis
- My father had Myasthenia Gravis

So, for years, I sought a diagnosis of my condition. For years, my parents stood by me, helping me when I needed it, loving my children and being surrogates when they needed them, and fighting with me for an understanding of what was happening to me.

They had seen me through knee surgeries and miscarriage. They saw me through divorce and loss. They saw me through every single challenge and rejoiced at every single triumph.

Then, one horrible summer, we lost both of them. It's been more than ten years and I miss them no less. So, here I was, in need of my mom's hug and my father's strong hands wrapped around mine, and I felt that loss as keenly as ever.

Suddenly, there were his words on a page. There was his voice in my head. As I retyped his composition for this book, I could hear him, smell his Old Spice, and feel him beside me. If I ever had any doubt of where I get my ideals, reading his words cleared that up for me:

"The Killer Within"
Richard M. Austin
1996
(edited only for publication purposes)

My initial response on hearing the diagnosis was "Anything that begins with mys..., has two words, and ends with gravis sounds kind of ominous". But then you have to understand that this was a reaction from someone who usually saw his doctor once a year for his annual physical and left the office with the doctor saying, "I'll see you next year" and that's when he would.

At sixty-seven years, the idea of death does not frighten me. It is an honest realization of where I am in life, as compared to the perception of immortality at, say, twenty-seven. The only part of dying that is scary, is the prospect of being sick with a long drown-out battle with a debilitating disease that robs you of the capability to live as you have been used to doing. That was the reason for the outburst on first learning what I had.

Ever since I was sixty-three, and had outlived my father who had died at that age, I have tried to look at each day granted me as a bonus and use it in such a way that, at the day's end, I could feel as if it had been worthwhile. The statistical rate of success might be questionable, but doing things that way at least gave living a direction. Now that I know I cohabit my body with something that can challenge my ability to maintain that ideal, I feel it is even more imperative to appreciate the positives in my life and exploit them to the fullest.

Some years ago, while preparing a Sunday School lesson, I came across an anecdote about an old man (I'm not there yet), who was asked to reflect on his life and how he would see it in retrospect. He answered the question by saying that he saw it as if he were standing on a hilltop at sunset, looking out over a vast landscape of hills and valleys, with the valleys deep in shadow and the hilltops still brightly gleaming in the sun.

All the details of the valleys were lost in the shadows, while the high points were still clear and vivid. What a glorious way to look at a life. But then the Lord gave us a short memory for pain and isn't that what we might expect? I hope that if I am ever old and am asked that question, my answer might be on the same level. What a terrible disappointment it must be to look back over the years that you have lived and wonder what the worth of it all is.

The fact of the matter is that I have been a much-blessed man throughout my life. As I mention earlier, my health has always been good, except for the usual aches and pains and sniffles. I have never even suffered a broken bone. I have loved and been loved by a wonderful woman for forty-six years, who even now serves as an inspiration in handling my first real physical adversity, because she has two of the same types of diseases and handles them with such courage.

One thing you can say about my family is when we get sick we never get ordinary things. We tend to collect rare diseases, thereby giving life an even more unique challenge. Money has always been a problem, but even there we're are able to get by as a one-income family, which we felt gave us a much better family life, despite the emotional stress that occasionally cropped up.

My children were a miracle in their own time, for various reasons, and have continued to bless us with our grandchildren and with their continuing care and concern. We have been surrounded with friends, find continuing spiritual fulfillment and sustenance in our church, live in an albeit small home that provides a haven for our life and friendly neighbors. A professionally-prepared net worth analysis might take issue with the idea – but I am an extremely wealthy man in every way that really counts.

This being the situation, how can I say that my life is over? I can't and I won't. My roommate in my body is just going to have to realize that, on any given day, he might be in command, but his tenure will be short-lived. When I was diagnosed and the disease named, my son "came up on the internet" and got me more information than I really wanted to know.

One of the things that was said was that a person with Myasthenia Gravis can live a "normal life". I know that a patient's idea of a normal life and that of a doctor can frequently diverge widely. A doctor might feel that, as long as you're breathing, eating and somewhat mobile, you are living normally. That does not take into account that many little things the patient has done for years he or she can now no longer do. It is the situation of a still sharp and active mind realizing the limitations that have been placed on their body and the frustration that accompanies that awareness. The sense of being trapped in a failing vessel and the feeling of being diminished by it. My hope and prayer is that the years I have tried to treat my time as bonus time will help me keep that sense of frustration at bay, so that I can feel that I will still be able to look at the end of each day with satisfaction and look forward to those yet to be granted.

When I was fifty-five years old, I used to tell people that I wished I could retire then and take on full-time the list of personal projects I had already made up. I figured even then I would have to live to be one hundred years old to complete it without adding anything. I retired at sixty-five without completing any of that list and adding enough to have to go to one hundred and fifty. I don't have time for frustration and self-pity. There is too much joy and satisfaction left to achieve. There is even a greater sense of urgency, in a good way, to make the most of what God has left to give me.

I cannot thank my sister enough for sharing this with me, at the moment I needed it most. I cannot thank my father enough for writing it all down and leaving us with the legacy of his words and his spirit, and for reminding me of just where I come from, from the strong stock, deep roots, and uplifting wings that bore me.

Like my father, I choose to focus on this

glorious life and never doubt the worth of any of it. And like both my mother and father, I feel there is far too much to do, too much joy and satisfaction left to achieve, to let a chronic illness steal any of that away from me.

Living our truth

This chapter is a risk and I know that going in. Why is it a risk? Because I'm going to talk about something outside the mainstream, as I did with soul loss earlier. I hope you will read it and let it sink in and consider, just consider, what I'm saying.

There are many of us who suffered abuse at an early age. Others who were taught to keep in and hide strong emotions, for one reason or another. As teens and adults, we suffered more abuse and kept more inside. It is a cycle that is often reinforced and repeated.

Looking back over fifty-four years, I can see the cycles of my illness corresponding to the cycles of the emotional and physical abuse I suffered. Add in traumatic illnesses and you have an almost lethal mix.

We are coming back to the recognition of our inherent mind-body connections, something previous civilizations saw clearly but something we have dismissed over a few centuries. How we ever discounted this connection is beyond me, but we humans are masters at denying our instincts and our inner workings.

According to recent studies, women who experience three types of trauma or adversity s children or teens had a sixty percent greater risk of experiencing autoimmune disease as adults. I have no doubt that extreme stress is a trigger for whatever this 'neurological disease' is with which I live. It is this very soul loss I wrote of earlier in this book. It is only when we are fully ourselves, living a life that is true to ourselves, that we can find true health, wellness, and wholeness.

It's not only me. I have known many people, particularly women, who have the same legacy and live with chronic illnesses, diagnosed and undiagnosed. And while Western medicine will tell you that stress does not trigger illness, I know few who live with it who would agree.

Why we don't see the connection is beyond me. We know the havoc that stress causes in our bodies, disrupting almost all of our bodies' processes. We know that living in extremely stressful situations keeps our cortisol levels high enough to do real damage. We also know it alters autoimmune responses. Long term, why couldn't it alter all this permanently?

I'm not saying everyone with chronic illness has been abused or lived in extremely stressful situations for long periods of time, and is sick as a result. I *am* saying that I have, and I believe there is a connection.

Perhaps the stress turns on the switch, that I was predisposed for to begin with. Or perhaps it has altered enough in my body to allow the illness to take hold. Either way, I see a connection, and I am merely suggesting you take a look to see if this is true for you as well.

I am *not* saying it's all in our heads. I'm saying our 'heads', our hearts, our souls, and our bodies are so interconnected and so interdependent that what happens to one, happens to all.

I'm only just learning to follow extreme stress with periods of down time, to relax and reassess and return to myself. Because I have trouble breathing, I now take a few days to focus on deep breathing and meditation. I seek solitude and intense quiet (that is a real thing for me) to silence the stress and reduce the adrenaline and cortisol.

I visualize my lungs filling easily and my blood brightening with oxygen, my heart beating at a slow and healthy pace. I visualize my organs in a relaxed and normal state and my blood pressure at peaceful levels. I see myself, body and soul, as calm and silent and at peace. And, of course, I write. As Jean-Luc Picard would say, I make it so.

This process silences the demons of stress

and returns me to a centered and grounded state. It not only allows me to calm; it also allows me to clearly see the lessons in the chaos.

Another source of body-altering stress is not having good personal boundaries. I wrote about this elsewhere in the book, but it is something worth revisiting because it is part and parcel to not living a life true to yourself.

Whether because of abuse or neglect or learning from others around us, many of us have no personal boundaries. We let others take and take and take from us. We offer our help and our time and our energy to others endlessly. We let others intrude into our personal lives and personal space. And, if we do manage to squeak out a 'no' now and then, we eat ourselves up inside with guilt.

People with strong personal boundaries give of themselves, of their time, and of their talents. The difference is that they set limits because they recognize that they need to refill the well from time to time. Just as writers must set strong boundaries around the precious time allotted to them to write, all of us need to do the same with time for ourselves.

This time, this stepping aside to regroup and refresh, is not selfish, though many of us (parents in particular) have been taught that it is. Everyone needs downtime. Everyone needs time to themselves. And, let's face it, we all need to miss one another now and then, to appreciate the time we do spend together.

Chronic illness offers you the gift of allowing you to assess and evaluate and then choose what to do and what not to do. While it should not preclude you from living your life, it does afford the kind of boundary that allows you to value time to yourself, time alone with loved ones, and time to create the life you want to be living.

And, so, here is Fred again. I knocked him out once and I will do so again. Because, I find that when I compromise the truth of who I am, when I allow myself to be sucked into that world of compromising who I am and self-editing to please other people, Fred gains ground. That won't be happening again.

Just as I do when editing a manuscript, I looked for the real story when the doctor made his pronouncement. I chipped away at what I don't need, to get to the heart of what lies beneath.

Somewhere under all the anger and dismay was the heart of the matter, beating softly. This is yet another chance to leave behind all that is not me, and to re-emerge more authentic, more congruent, and more true to who I really am. Now, it's not 'their' truth I'm living; it's mine. And it's up to me to make it a masterpiece.

So, here we are at the end of the book and

the beginning of a new chapter for me. Stay tuned! My story continues, and I am once again getting reacquainted with myself. I intend to keep fighting, even as I reclaim who I am. I hope you will keep fighting, too.

Epilogue: Monster Slayer

A sword, like a statue found within a block of marble, is found within cold, hard, ugly iron. There is no sign of what lies within, when only looking at the fodder brought to the smith.

The iron is forged in the intense heat of a blacksmith's fire to make it malleable. It is folded and beaten again and again, in a long process that must be done just so. The final tensile strength and the lethal edge come from this process. Too fast and the sword would be brittle and break. Too slow and it will not be finished.

The perfect sword must be strong, flexible, sharp, and well-balanced. It takes a master to create such a weapon. It takes a master to wield one effectively and efficiently. These masters study a lifetime to hone their craft, making mistakes and moving on to learn from them, to do better the next time.

Those of us living with chronic illnesses are being forged in a fire of pain and challenge. We are being folded and beaten and melted on a daily basis. We are being tested and tried. We are being honed and sharpened. We fall, we fail, we weep, we rail against our own bodies, and then we wake up and do it all again the next day. We, too, learn and move on.

Through it all, we are like the butterfly emerging from a dark night of the soul in its cocoon. As Sam experiences in my story *Love in the Middle*, the stuff we were made of has been destroyed, disintegrated, demolished. What emerges is made of the same stuff but is transformed into a thing of grace and beauty. Yet, as much as I love the butterfly analogy, I prefer to think we are more like the phoenix.

Like a phoenix, our transformation may occur more than once. There is a lesson to be learned each time, and strength and wisdom to be gained. Unlike the phoenix, we can choose to learn and grow… or not.

It would do us all well to remember we are made of both earth and stardust, just as a sword is made of steel and fire, because we are grounded in our Earth Mother, as well as sisters and brothers of the stars. We are Spirits unchained, merely borrowing these fragile bodies we now carry with us. And, Spirit is unbreakable.

This is not the end.
There is no end.
There is only transformation.

Appendices

Recipes to get you started

Unless otherwise stated, all ingredients should be raw and certified organic. Most recipes require only a blender and a sharp knife. While the vegetable 'pasta' is best prepared from a spiral slicer, a sharp knife and some patience will get you started.

It only takes moments to prepare a simple meal. I can juice four apples (about one cup of juice) to drink, and warm water enough to melt miso paste and slice some mushrooms, scallions and tofu to add to my 'soup' in only a matter of minutes. Certainly as simple as making a sandwich and brewing a cup of coffee. Don't be daunted by the idea of eating raw!

Remember to adapt any recipes you use to your taste. Garlic, hot peppers, and spices provide warmth that you may feel is lacking by not cooking your food. And, be certain to rotate your ingredients and your menus. Not only will this keep you from getting bored with your meals, it will keep your body in top condition.

Raw plant fats are seeds, nuts, avocado, olives, and coconuts. These fats are soft, heavy, and filling, so they fill the empty spaces and ground you, bringing you back to earth. They satisfy hunger. They feed your nerves, so you're happier and handle stress with a smile. Seed and nut milks are a delicious way to eat fats,

Raw fruits are all foods with seeds for their own propagation. They include the sweet fruits we love, plus sour fruits (cranberry, grapefruit, lemon, lime), vegetable fruits (bell pepper, cucumber, okra, pumpkin, squash, tomato, zucchini), and sun-dried fruits. Try to eat only red or yellow peppers, not green peppers (they're less ripe, which is why they can 'repeat' on you).

Raw greens should ideally be living, to harness the healing and energy within. That means, eat them as close to picking time as possible, preferably from your own bed of growing greens.

Several recipes in this chapter include germinated nuts, beans or seeds. Germinating these foods before you eat them releases all their nutrients and energy. To eat them simply raw is to miss out on all they have to offer. Eating all grown food as close to harvest offers that much more energy and nutrients as well.

To germinate organic raw nuts, beans or seeds:
1. Rinse the raw nuts, beans or seeds and then soak them in room-temperature filtered water for the proper amount of time (usually 3-4 hours depending on the nut) in a clean glass jar. Cover with cheesecloth or an old stocking.
2. When done, drain and rinse with filtered water a few times. I prefer to use a colander and toss them about a bit as I rinse them. You can now eat them as is or use them in any of the following recipes.

To sprout organic beans or seeds (after you've germinated them):
1. Place germinated seeds or beans in a sprouting container, making sure they are well-drained and ventilated. Cover with cheesecloth or old stocking to keep bugs out.
2. Set the sprouting container on your counter and allow the beans or seeds to sprout for the required amount of time.
3. Rinse with filtered water several times and drain well.
4. Sprouts can be eaten up to five days later, if stored in an air-tight container in your refrigerator. It helps to have two or more jars going, so you always have fresh sprouts on hand.

Kitchen add-ons:

You don't need to purchase anything new, as far as appliances and gadgets to make these changes in your lifestyle, but there are some that really help. Anything that helps you out, makes things easier, and makes this transition simpler for you is always worth considering.

Blender: A really good, powerful blender helps with smoothies and fresh soups. Having a smoothie cup attachment saves transferring your delicious drink into another glass and then having to wash two!

Spiralizer or spiral slicer: Once you get hooked on making fresh veggie "pasta", this gadget will be your best friend. Most are very straightforward to use and clean.

Dehydrator: These come in all shapes, sizes, and price ranges. If you're interested in trying one, I suggest searching your local 'trash and treasure' group on FB, as people often buy them and then never use them. Be sure to get the additional non-stick sheets for your trays, so that you can make things like fruit leathers and 'sun-dried' tomatoes. And, it is a great way to preserve all that amazing organic produce you grow (or purchase at the farmer's market).

Mandolin slicer: Great to have on hand, for larger, flatter slices. Definitely need one of these to make raw taco shells! (see recipe)

1 cup germinated almonds or other germinated nuts of your choice
2 cups pure water
1 tablespoon raw honey

Blend germinated almonds and water until almonds are pulverized. Strain and discard the solids in your compost pile. Blend the liquid with honey. Store in an airtight container in the refrigerator.

Note: you can strain the liquid through cheesecloth or even 'nutmilk bags'. I use the small linen bags available at craft stores. I turn them inside out to get all the 'pulp' (which I use in dehydrated cookies) and then launder them for reuse.

3 cups whole organic oats
½ cup organic raisins or dried cranberries or dried blueberries
1 cup germinated almonds or other nuts
½ cup sprouted seeds
½ cup ground organic flax seed
Several teaspoons ground cinnamon, to taste
Raw honey

Warm the oatmeal in a frying pan over low heat. Transfer to a glass bowl and drizzle honey over the warm oats and mix together. Add honey until it is all coated. Lightly chop the germinated almonds in blender. Toss oats with the raisins, cinnamon and chopped nuts. Put in airtight container, as is, let cool and then cover. Eat with a dash of raw nut milk or over non-fat yogurt and fresh fruit, for a great breakfast, or, as is, as a snack.

Or, substitute organic low-fat vanilla yogurt for the honey, spread out about 1/2" thick on liner sheets and score into bars. Place into dehydrator until firm and cut into bars.

2 teaspoons unpasteurized miso paste
2 teaspoons liquid aminos
2 cups filtered water
¼-1/2 sheet dried seaweed, torn or cut into bite-size pieces
One handful sliced raw mushrooms, scallions, or other raw veggies of your choice
Diced extra-firm tofu

Mix the miso with liquid aminos. Heat the water only enough to dissolve the miso paste (but do not boil) and pour it over the miso and Bragg mixture and stir until completely dissolved. Add more Bragg Liquid Aminos if you'd like the broth to be saltier. Add the seaweed and mushrooms, scallions, and tofu, letting them warm and soften. Makes two servings. Excellent with some dehydrated crackers for lunch or dinner!

6 large tomatoes, diced
½ red onion, chopped
1 bell pepper, seeded and diced
2 cloves garlic, mined
1 cucumber, chopped
Pure water
3 tablespoons apple cider vinegar
One lemon
4 tablespoons chopped fresh cilantro
Sea Salt to taste
1 scallion, chopped

Place the tomatoes, onion, pepper, garlic, and cucumber in your blender. Add the freshly squeezed juice from the lemon, the vinegar and the cilantro. Puree well, making sure all the pieces are reduced to a pulpy mixture. Add water and sea salt to taste and to improve mixture, blending on low one last time. Chill until quite cold and sprinkle the scallions over the soup before serving.

¼ c. cold-pressed olive oil
2 tablespoons liquid aminos
¼ c. raw apple cider vinegar
4" fresh ginger root, grated
¼ lemon, squeezed
½ teaspoon organic miso paste

Combine all ingredients in a blender and liquify. Toss into a fresh salad or toss fresh veggies in dressing before stacking on a slice of sprouted bread for an open-faced sandwich. I also love raw vegetables toss in this dressing and rolled into a flatbread for a savory breakfast.
Also good on grilled salmon.

3 cups germinated chickpeas
1 cup cold-pressed olive oil
½ cup raw organic tahini, stirred to blend
2 cloves garlic, minced
Juice of ½ lemon, freshly squeezed
Filtered water
Sea salt to taste

Puree the germinated chickpeas in blender with ½ cup of the oil. Add water slowly to reach desired consistency (thick but completely pulverized). When creamy, add tahini, garlic and lemon juice. Keep blending until smooth and creamy. Add sea salt to taste. Can be eaten immediately, but I find that it improves when you chill it in the refrigerator overnight.

Great with sprouted crackers, spread over sprouted bread and topped with raw sliced veggies, or on top of greens as a salad.

And you can take hummus beyond chickpeas! Try edamame, lima beans, black beans, green peas, beets, squash, kale, spinach, sweet potatoes, and more. Check out the next recipe for another delicious alternative...

1 (24-ounce) can white beans, drained and rinse completely
2 lemons, juiced
1 teaspoon ground cumin (you can add more to taste)
2 garlic cloves, minced
1/2 cup tahini paste
1/2 cup cold-pressed, extra-virgin olive oil
Sea salt

Put all ingredients in a food-processor or heavy-duty blender and process until smooth and creamy. Sample it and add salt to taste. Blend again and then refrigerate. While you can eat it right away, I find the taste improves even more when it is refrigerated overnight.

I love this as a dip with raw vegetables, as well as spread on sprouted grain toast and topped with sliced heirloom tomatoes or avocado. It can also be spread on lavash and topped with thinly-sliced raw vegetables and then rolled and sliced in half.

5 large heirloom tomatoes, diced small (liquid drained)
1 bell pepper, diced small
½ red onion, diced small
2 cloves garlic, minced
1 small 'hot' pepper, finely chopped and seeded (choose one that suits your favored level of heat, and remember the hotter the pepper, the more careful you have to be handling it.)
¼ cup fresh cilantro, finely chopped
¼ cup cold-pressed olive oil
Sea salt to taste

Combine all ingredients, tossing together well, until fully blended. Flavor with sea salt to taste. Can be eaten immediately, but I find that it improves when you chill it in the refrigerator overnight. Enjoy with sprouted crackers or with chicken or fish to enhance a meal.

Refrigerate and use within a day or two of making. I find refrigerating overnight helps blend the flavors better.

I love to use different kinds of heirloom tomatoes, to get a real depth of flavor and color. You can mix this up by adding finely diced raw mango or peaches, to add a sweetness to your salsa

4 cups whole flax seeds, soaked 4-6 hours
1/3 to 1/2 cup liquid aminos
2 lemons, juiced
Spices of your choice
Filtered water

Soak flax seeds for 4 to 6 hours in filtered water. You will then have a pasty mixture, be sure to keep moist and loose for spreading. Add aminos, spices and lemon juice to taste and mix well. Spread mixture as thin as possible on your dehydrator trays with a liner sheet on top. Keep your hands wet as this will help on spreading the flax seeds (or use a spatula). Dehydrate at 105 degrees for 5-6 hours and then flip the mixture on the liner sheet. Continue dehydrating until the mixture completely dry. Approximately 5-6 hours.

Chia seeds make a similar 'paste' that you can try, as well. Try adding in some sesame seeds for an extra nutty flavor or sprinkle with real, freshly-grated parmesan cheese before dehydrating.

1 pkg. gravlox marinated salmon, chopped
1 tomato, finely chopped
¼ red onion, finely chopped
1 tsp. fresh dill or oregano, finely chopped
1 tsp. apple cider vinegar
1 tsp. cold-pressed olive oil
2 cups raw baby spinach

Combine all ingredients until well mixed and then mound over fresh baby spinach or a kale/spinach/Brussel sprout 'super salad' mix. Also great on top of gluten-free parmesan crackers or my flax seed crackers.

I also love to top my flax crackers with small pieces of gravlox and add a salad, for an easy, tasty meal that keeps me going during the day.

1 medium-sized yellow summer squash or zucchini

Slice the squash very thin with a very sharp knife or use a spiral slicer to create exceptionally thin 'pasta'. Top with raw sauce of your choice.

Pesto Sauce
(single serving)

½ cup cold pressed olive oil
½ cup pine nuts
1 cup fresh basil, chopped
1 clove garlic, minced
¼ lemon, squeezed
Sea salt, to taste

Combine all ingredients in a blender and puree. Toss squash 'pasta' with sauce and serve immediately. For a nice variation on this recipe, use lemon basil to add a nice lemony taste.

Tomato Sauce

(single serving)
2 large tomatoes, sliced
1 clove of garlic
Fresh basil, chopped
Fresh oregano, chopped
¼ red onion, sliced

2 tablespoons cold pressed olive oil
½ lemon, squeezed
Sea salt to taste

Combine all ingredients in a blender and puree. Let sit for a few moments to thicken. Toss squash 'pasta' with sauce and serve immediately. Add some hot pepper to add 'heat' if desired.

Finely chopped raw mushrooms
A very small dash of olive oil
Pinch of lime salt
Ground cumin to taste
Jicama root, peeled
Taco toppings of choice including chopped heirloom tomatoes, onion, cilantro, cheese, etc.

Use a mandolin slicer to create very thin jicama 'taco shells'. These will be nice and crunchy. You can toast lightly if you want to remove some of the moisture.

Mix the first three ingredients and spoon into jicama shells. Top with your toppings of choice and enjoy!

Raw sweet potato or peeled jicama, sliced to ¼" slices
Toppings of choice including raw nut butters, smashed potatoes, berries, sliced bananas, nuts, and other options

Place sliced sweet potato or jicama in toaster. For sweet potatoes, toast twice. I toast jicama three times on a setting of "4" to get out some of the moisture. Then top with toppings of choice and enjoy!

3 lbs. firm eggplant (about 3 medium eggplants)
2 yellow onions (or 1 medium), chopped finely
3 gloves garlic, minced
1 tablespoon olive oil
1 teaspoon sea salt
1½ lbs. tahini
1 lemon, squeezed
3 cups water
1 cup nama shoyu or tamari sauce
Cayenne pepper, to taste

Cut eggplant thinly lengthwise. Marinate in water, nama shoyu or tamari sauce and ½ teaspoon sea salt for at least 2 hours, and up to 12 hours. Dry the eggplant slices with a paper towel.

Process or chop eggplant, onions, garlic, tahini, lemon juice, remaining salt and a pinch of cayenne pepper until very finely chopped and mixed. Serve over greens or with sprouted crackers.

1 large bunch of fresh spinach
1 handful of raw pine nuts
1-2 teaspoons of coconut oil
Juice of one fresh lemon
1 sheet of lavash (it comes in very large sheets, but I use the smaller pre-cut sheets)
Additional ingredients as desired (sweet hot pepper spread, sliced tomatoes, etc.)

Puree the spinach, pine nuts, coconut oil, and lemon juice, until it's a fairly smooth paste. Spread one quarter of the puree over the sheet of lavash. Store the rest in the refrigerator.

Next, spread a little sweet hot pepper spread over the puree, or place evenly-spaced, thinly sliced heirloom tomatoes, or another topping of your choice.

Roll the lavash and slice down the middle. Eat immediately or refrigerate for a power lunch.

When you eat nourishing food and drink a lot of water, your will find that your body changes may include better-looking skin, as well as feeling more energy and less lethargy. Internal changes for the better can begin to show in your eyes, your hair, your skin... which in turn, make you feel better about what you're doing and improve how you feel about yourself in general. There are, in addition, changes you can make externally, too!

Again, this is just to get you started. There are great recipes for alternative laundry detergent (to element waxes and chemicals from your clothing). Vinegar is an amazing fabric softener and is a healthy alternative for anyone who lives with skin issues or has very sensitive skin. Felted dryer balls also work great to soften and eliminate static in your dryer. All natural and all healthier for you.

Another benefit of using all-natural ingredients is that they are good for the world around you. Nothing bad going back into our groundwater, less plastic going into our landfills, and no animals harmed by either testing or disposal of any of these products. Doesn't that make you feel better already?

I have experienced a lot of changes in my skin, from illness, medications, and age. I love coconut oil mixed with a little baking soda as a facial scrub.

1 ramekin of coconut oil
1 Tb baking soda

I keep it in a wee ramekin in my bathroom, apply with light touch before my shower, and let the hot, moist air work on it while I wash my hair and body. I rinse it off at the end of my shower, and my skin feels smooth and actually nourished! I have also started applying just coconut oil to my face and any dry patches of skin, during the day, and can feel a huge difference since starting that regime. Plus, no worries about additives or animal testing.

There is a lot of talk about aluminum and its possible link to breast cancer or Alzheimer's. While I cannot speak to the validity of that claim, I do think it makes sense not to take those kinds of chances with our bodies, especially when there are healthy alternatives.

1 ramekin of coconut oil
1 Tb baking soda
1 Tb arrowroot powder
Essential oils or ground herbs (optional)

Mix baking soda and arrowroot together in a small bowl.
Blend in coconut oil. This is easier if the oil is slightly warm and more liquid than solid.
Add 2-3 drops essential oils, if desired, or ground dried mint, lavender, etc and add to oil mixture.
Store in small glass jar or ramekin.
Apply small amount under arms daily.

Note: Be sure that you test this (and any topical skin care products) on a very small patch of skin (inside of your wrist works well for this) to be sure there is no reaction. Do not use too much essential oil, as it can case dermatitis, especially in such a warm, sensitive area as an armpit.

Other books and websites to help you get started

(Please note: none of the listings below are paid endorsements. These are books and sites that I have used and that I feel might get you off to a good start. All are available as of the time this book goes to press, unless otherwise noted)

Referenced books:

* Elizabeth Kubler-Ross, *On Grief and Grieving: Finding the Meaning Through the Five Stages of Loss* (Scribner, 2014)
* Seth King, *Honesty,* 2016 (CreateSpace)

Raw Food Diet and Overcoming Illness with Food

* Susan Irby, *The Bikini Chef® Diet,* www.thebikinichef.com
* Susan Irby, *Boost Your Metabolism,* www.thebikinichef.com
* Carol Alt, *Eating in the Raw: A Beginner's Guide to Getting Slimmer, Feeling Healthier, and Looking Younger the Raw-Food Way* (Clarkson Potter, 2010)
* Alisa Cohen, *Living on Live Food* (Cohen Publishing, 2004, out of print but available through third-party sellers)
* Steve Meyerowitz, *Sproutman's Kitchen Garden Cookbook* (Sproutman Publications, 1999)

* James Levin and Natalie Cederquist, *Vibrant Living* by (Glo, 2001, out of print but available through third-party sellers)

* Growing and Using Herbs
* Louise Riotte, *Rodale's Illustrated Encyclopedia of Herbs*
* Louise Riotte, *Carrots Love Tomatoes: Secrets of Companion Planting for Successful Gardening*, 2nd edition. 1998. (Storey Communications)
* Louise Riotte, *Roses Love Garlic: Companion Planting and Other Secrets of Flowers*. 1998. (Storey Communications)
* H. Philbrick and R. Gregg, *Companion Plants and, How to Use Them*. 1966. (Devin-Adair Publishers)
* Jack R. Pyle and Taylor Reese, *Raising with The Moon: The Complete Guide to Gardening and Living by the Signs of the Moon*. 1993. (Down Home Press, Asheboro, NC.)

Meditation, Visualization, Celtic Spirituality, Ecopsychology, and Reconnecting with the Earth
* John Matthews, *The Celtic Shaman*. 2001, (Rider & Co., out of print but available through third-party sellers
* David Abram, *The Spell of the Sensuous*. 1997. (Vintage)
* Frank MacEowen, *The Mist-Filled Path: Celtic*

Wisdom for Exiles, Wanderers, and Seekers. 2002. (New World Library)

* Frank MacEowen, *The Spiral of Memory and Belonging: A Celtic Path of Soul and Kinship* (New World Library, 2004)

* *Yearning for the Wind: Celtic Reflections on Nature and Soul* by Tom Gowan, 2003 (New World Library)

* Thich Nhat Hanh. *The Miracle of Mindfulness: An Introduction to the Practice of Meditation,* 1996. (Beacon Press)

* Ken Carey, *Return of the Bird Tribes,* 2011 (Harper Collins)

Shamanism and Soul-Retrieval

* Bill Plotkin, *Soulcraft: Crossing into the Mysteries of Nature and Psyche,* 2010 (New World Library)

* Caitlin Matthews, *Singing the Soul Back Home: Shamanic Wisdom for Every Day,* 2003. (Connections Book Publishing)

* Jeannette Gagan, *Journeying: Where Shamanism and Psychology Meet,* 1998 (Rio Chama Publications)

* Sandra Ingerman, *Soul Retrieval: Mending the Fragmented Self,* 1998. (HarperOne)

* Serge Kahili King, *Urban Shaman~ A handbook for personal and planetary transformation based on the Hawaiian way of the Adventurer,* 1990. (Touchstone)

* Michael Samuels and Mary Rockwood Lane, *Shaman Wisdom, Shaman Healing: Deepen Your Ability to Heal with Visionary and Spiritual Tools and Practices*, 2008. (Wiley)

Art as Healing

* Pat B. Allen, *Art is a Spiritual Path: Engaging the Sacred through the Practice of Art and Writing* by *Art is a Way of Knowing*, 2013 (Shambhala Publications)
* Michael Samuels, *Healing with the Mind's Eye: How to Use Guided Imagery and Visions to Heal Mind, Body, and Spirit*, 2003. (Wiley)
* Michael Samuels and Mary Rockwood Lane, *Creative Healing: How to Heal Yourself by Tapping Your Hidden Creativity*, 1998. (John Wiley and Sons)
* Michell Cassou and Stewart Cubley, *Life, Paint, and Passion: Reclaiming the Magic of Spontaneous Expression,* 2000. (Jeremy P. Tarcher)
* Shaun McNiff, *Art as Medicine*, 1992. (Shambhala)
* Julia Cameron, *The Artist's Way*, 2002. (Jeremy P. Tarcher/Putnam)

Websites:

* Heather Plett, *What It Really Means to Hold Space for Someone*, 2016. www.upliftconnect.com/hold-space/ (quoted with permission)
* Christine Miserandino, *The Spoon Theory*, www.butyoudontlooksick.com/articles/written-by-christine/the-spoon-theory/
* Beautiful 'Thrive' Spoon pendants, by Phoenix Magyk. http://phoenixmagyk.com/
* Eden Organic Nursery, www.eonseed.com, for organic seeds and more
* Notes from the Universe, www.tut.com, for daily inspirational messages tailored to your personal goals.

About the Author

Barbara Lieberman's stories are about the power of words, the power of love, and the consequences of the choices we make. They range from fairy tales illustrated children's books, from an historical fiction series to historical romance. and, now, non-fiction. She is a partner in Pipe & Thimble Publishing with her daughter, Ellie Lieberman.

A New Jersey native, Barbara moved to beautiful Southern California in 2012 to start over yet again. A mother of two amazing young adults, an avid gardener, a life-long (and long-suffering) Phillies fan, and a voracious reader, Barbara is also one of the many people living with an undiagnosed neurological illness.

*Voted one of the 50 Great Writers You Should Be Reading for 2015
The Treasure of Ravenwood: A Fairy Tale by Barbara Lieberman has been voted to the top 40 Best Chapter Books for Young Girls List on Goodreads.
The Treasure of Ravenwood. Ben's Little Acorn and *Why Does the Moon Follow Me?* are Reading Is Fundamental books and Barbara is proud to be a RIF Author Partner.

You can find the author at:
FB: bliebermanauthor
Twitter: Seeds2Inspire
Website: www.keyboardmusings.com

Unchaining Your Spirit: Living with Chronic Illness is a companion book that helps you chart your challenges and track your triumphs. I know first-hand that living with chronic illness can be both a challenge and a blessing. Some days, you win the Nobel Prize; some days, you do the laundry. The pages inside offer you a new way to focus on your life, so that you can truly live well, rather than just existing within the cloud of illness.

Based on **The Unchained Spirit.**

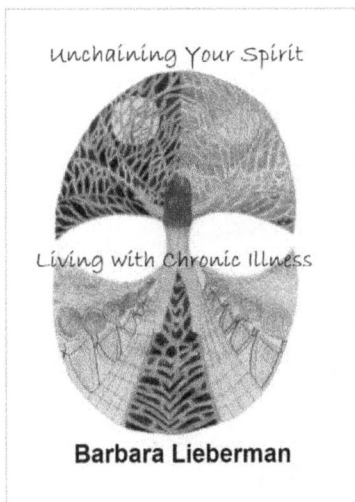

unchaining Your Spirit

Living with Chronic Illness

Barbara Lieberman

Available on Amazon, Barnes & Noble, and other online retailers, as well as the author's website: www.keyboardmusings.com